PUBLIC HEALTH IN THE 21ST CENTURY

ACTIVITIES OF DAILY LIVING (ADL)

CULTURAL DIFFERENCES, IMPACTS OF DISEASE AND LONG-TERM HEALTH EFFECTS

PUBLIC HEALTH IN THE 21ST CENTURY

Additional books in this series can be found on Nova's website
under the Series tab.

Additional e-books in this series can be found on Nova's website
under the e-book tab.

PUBLIC HEALTH IN THE 21ST CENTURY

ACTIVITIES OF DAILY LIVING (ADL)

CULTURAL DIFFERENCES, IMPACTS OF DISEASE AND LONG-TERM HEALTH EFFECTS

SCOTT T. LIVELY
EDITOR

New York

Library of Congress Cataloging-in-Publication Data

ISBN: 978-1-63463-913-2
Library of Congress Control Number: 2014960312

Published by Nova Science Publishers, Inc. † New York

Contents

Preface

Alzheimer's disease (AD) is a debilitating neurodegenerative disease which commonly occurs later in life. In the early stages of AD, everyday tasks such as making a cup of coffee, managing finances and other tasks which require complex interaction with the environment, become difficult for an individual to perform. These tasks facilitate independent living and quality of life, and are referred to as Instrumental Activities of Daily Living (IADL). However, as this disease progresses, even basic activities of daily living (BADL), such as bathing, toileting and eating meals, which are fundamental to self-care, become difficult to carry out unaided. This book examines the cognitive and neural correlation AD has on ADL. Furthermore, the book discusses the quality of life of patients with knee osteoarthritis; real-time fall detection systems that aim for fall prevention; disability and ethnicities; hand functionality during activities of daily living; and rehabilitation strategies used to promote independence in daily living tasks for people with cognitive impairments.

Chapter 1 – During the course of Alzheimer's disease and other types of dementia, patients develop cognitive and neuropsychiatric impairments, which increase in severity. These deficits impact their ability to perform everyday tasks, which leads to lower quality of life and loss of independence. This chapter contains a summary of the methods used to study activities of daily living (ADL) in patients with dementia. Associated information will be provided on the cognitive processes which are related to reductions in ADL. Much of the neuroimaging research has focused on identifying the brain regions that are subject to atrophy due to different pathologies, and on investigating the neural correlates of cognitive abilities such as memory. A much smaller number of functional and structural neuroimaging studies have been devoted specifically to identifying the brain regions that underpin functional abilities. This chapter will also review that literature, and will highlight the brain regions which are compromised when deficits in ADL are apparent. A more complete understanding of the neural underpinnings of functional abilities may enable more accurate prognosis and more effective interventions to be developed. The chapter will include suggestions for future directions for the study of ADL.

Chapter 2 – The incidence of age-related degenerative musculoskeletal disease is increasing in much of the industrialized world due to population aging. Knee osteoarthritis (OA) is one of the most common diseases in this category. Although not a disease that directly affects short-term survival, knee OA nonetheless negatively impacts essential activities of daily living (ADLs), activities parallel to daily living (APDLs), and general quality of life (QOL).Moreover, knee OA patients with limited mobility (sedentary) may be at greater risk of early mortality due to metabolic and cardiovascular diseases. First, this chapter discusses the prevalence of knee OA, the various diagnostic tools used, and the physical and psychological sequelae that influence disease-specific QOL. Second, the correlations among ADLs, APDLs, and disease-specific QOL are discussed. Finally, survey results on frequencies of disease-specific difficulties in ADLs (e.g., dressing the lower body, going to the toilet, and climbing stairs) and APDLs (e.g., cooking, washing, and cleaning) are presented. A significant fraction of knee OA patients who have maintained functional independence still experience difficulty with these daily tasks.

Chapter 3 – Falls are dangerous among the elderly population and are a major health concern. Many investigators and some commercial products have used accelerometers for real-time fall detection. Furthermore, the combination of miniature 3-D accelerometers and gyroscopes has also been used for fall detection sensors, but the effects of the optimal placement position of these sensors have not been studied thoroughly. Besides, intelligent algorithms can be used to improve the accuracy of these wearable fall detection sensors considerably. Therefore, in this chapter, the authorswill report two related fall detection studies that used slightly different sensor technologies and smart algorithms as follows: (1) the 1st study reports our custom-designed wired sensor (with both an accelerometer and two gyroscopes) placed as a single unit on three different positions along the thoracic vertebrae on subjects (i.e., T-4, T-7, and T-10). Results indicated that T-10 was not a good location for fall detection; however, both T-4 and T-7 were suitable, with the results for T-4 being slightly better. Using a simple rule-based multi-thresholds algorithm that utilizes the recorded resultant gravitational acceleration, angular change, angular velocity, and angular acceleration, the authorswere able to successfully detect all 60 falls and differentiate between falls and activities of daily living (ADL) with no false positives on young volunteers (note: backward falls were not included in this sensor placement study as the authorswere using a wired sensor). This naturally leads to our second study: (2) a real-time fall detection system using our improved *wireless* gait analysis sensor (WGAS) will be detailed. This WGAS is capable of differentiating falls vs. various Activities of Daily Living (ADL) and the Dynamic Gait Index (DGI) tests performed by young volunteers using a Back Propagation Artificial Neural Network (BP ANN) algorithm. The WGAS, which includes a tri-axial accelerometer, 2 gyroscopes, a wireless module and a Texas Instruments (TI) MSP430 microcontroller can be worn by the subjects at either T4 (at back) or on a belt-clip (in front at the center of the waist) for performing the various falls, ADL, and DGI tests. The raw gait data is wirelessly transmitted from the WGAS to a nearby PC for real-time fall classification, where six features were extracted for the BP ANN. Overall fall classification accuracies of 97.0% and 97.4% have been achieved for the data taken at the T4 and at the belt positions, respectively. The preliminary data demonstrates an overall sensitivity of 97.0% and overall specificity of 97.2% for this WGAS fall detection system, suggesting this can be a good candidate as a real-time low-cost and effective fall detection device for wireless acute-care and wireless assisted-living. The authorsare now collecting more clinical data using the WGAS system on both patients and volunteers for gait analysis targeting for fall prevention as well.

Chapter 4 – Disability in the elderly is a complex, dynamic and multidimensional condition. Recently, there has been a shift from an exclusively individual and medical perspective of disability to a new perspective which includes social-cultural factors. There is an interrelation between disability and functionality very similar to those that exist between health and disease. Disability has been linked to frailty, cognitive decline, higher prevalence of comorbidities, hospitalizations, mortality; impact in family life, stress, high costs, and health attention needs due to the increasing population of elderly. The WHO World Health Survey 2002-2004 reported a general worldwide prevalence of 38.1% in population 60 years or older, being higher in people of lower income countries, in women and in people who live in rural areas. Evaluation of disability is based on scales that report limitations of activities of daily living (ADL); these activities are divided into three sections: basic ADL, instrumental or intermediate ADL, and advanced ADLs. These instruments are widely used in diagnosing disability and in evaluating successful aging. However, there can be a great bias (if not corrected) that could influence the interpretation of its results: education and cultural differences. Activities of daily living are measured in a subjective way were the elderly usually self-report their results. Cultural differences influence in variation of results since activities of daily living are influenced by personal, family, and social perspective. Due to this self-report, some aged people may not inform the severity of their disability. An example of this issue is demonstrated in a prospective 6 year cohort study using the sample from the 1998 Health and Retirement Study studied how cultural and ethnic factors could affect the outcome of diagnosis in activities of daily living disability. Hispanics reported lower rates of walking disability even though higher frequencies of lower-extremity dysfunction were reported.

Another example could be a study that reported institutionalization due to limitations in ADLs in the Asian American elderly, where a smaller prevalence of institutionalization in Asian elderly was found compared to non-Hispanic white elderly. This result could be explained by the cultural difference that exists in the Asian elderly population. Asians are more collective than individualists, in other words, they prefer to seek help with family members instead of assisting for help in a nursing home. In conclusion, diagnosing disability is highly influenced by cultural differences. Lack of early diagnosis could in the end, affect prevalence of frailty, cognitive decline, comorbidities, and mortality in the elderly.

Chapter 5 – Over a billion people (about 15% of the world's population) are estimated to be living with some disability, according to the World Health Organization (WHO). To protect the human rights of people with disability, a great effort is being made to unify the classification of disabilities. The WHO's International Classification of Functioning, Disability and Health (ICF) has become a recognized reference for classifying the degree of disability. Beyond the obvious limitations derived from the lack of body functions and structures, the ability to carry out Activities of Daily Living (ADL) is proposed in the ICF as the main factor for classifying the degree of disability. According to the ICF, many of the deficiencies in the domains of activity and participation are focused on the upper limbs. Furthermore, hands are used for more than 5 hours a day only in ADL, excluding the time spent on working or sleeping. The functional evaluation of the hand in ADL is therefore essential to assess a person's degree of independence. Moreover, this evaluation is also important when it comes to examining the progress of rehabilitation programs or in clinical practice. At present, the functional evaluation of the hand is performed using qualitative methods like

"Disabilities of the Arm, Shoulder and Hand" (DASH), some of which are highly subjective and valid only for a specific pathology. Objective methods like measuring passive ranges of angles or maximal forces for specific types of grasps are also used, but no objective measurements while performing ADL are considered. No consensus has been reached about a unified method to assess hand functionality while performing ADL, as might be desirable, so that professionals have to rely on their own experience to grade this.

The aim of this chapter is to review the role of the use of the hand in the ability to perform ADL, with special attention given to the evaluations of functionality that are being used to establish the degree of disability and to monitor the evolution in rehabilitation processes for different pathologies of the hand. Special attention is paid to analyzing the attempts that have been made to objectify the evaluation of hand disabilities through the analysis of grasp and handling, and their impact on current practice.

Chapter 6 – In this chapter, rehabilitation strategies to promote independence in daily living tasks for people with cognitive impairments will be outlined. The clienteles described in this chapter include people after a stroke or brain injury, people with Parkinson's disease and mild cognitive impartment or dementia.

Two case reports using self-regulation and mental imagery respectively, one randomized clinical trial evaluating the effectiveness of a one-week self-regulation program and two randomized clinical trials on testing the efficacy of the three-week self-regulation and mental imagery interventions on post-stroke patients will be summarized in this paper. Mental imagery has been extended to be used by people with mild cognitive impairments. The strategy helps the people to maintain a perceptual map within which the daily tasks are structured. A clinical trial using rehabilitation strategies including mental imagery to promote cognitive function necessary for daily living task performance will be summarized in this chapter. The use of external aids is common for people with Parkinson's disease to help them in initiating motor performance. This treatment strategy is believed to arouse attention of the people in starting off the motor tasks. The use of external aids and how it is internalized using the treatment technique of mental imagery will be described. With the use of various rehabilitation strategies in the occupational therapy programs, people with cognitive impairment showed better performance of daily living tasks.

In: Activities of Daily Living (ADL)
Editor: Scott T. Lively

ISBN: 978-1-63463-913-2

Chapter 1

Activities of Daily Living in Alzheimer's Disease: Cognitive and Neural Correlates

Laura M. A. Kane and William J. McGeown*
School of Psychological Sciences and Health,
University of Strathclyde, UK

Abstract

During the course of Alzheimer's disease and other types of dementia, patients develop cognitive and neuropsychiatric impairments, which increase in severity. These deficits impact their ability to perform everyday tasks, which leads to lower quality of life and loss of independence. This chapter contains a summary of the methods used to study activities of daily living (ADL) in patients with dementia. Associated information will be provided on the cognitive processes which are related to reductions in ADL. Much of the neuroimaging research has focused on identifying the brain regions that are subject to atrophy due to different pathologies, and on investigating the neural correlates of cognitive abilities such as memory. A much smaller number of functional and structural neuroimaging studies have been devoted specifically to identifying the brain regions that underpin functional abilities. This

* Corresponding author: Email: william.mcgeown@strath.ac.uk

chapter will also review that literature, and will highlight the brain regions which are compromised when deficits in ADL are apparent. A more complete understanding of the neural underpinnings of functional abilities may enable more accurate prognosis and more effective interventions to be developed. The chapter will include suggestions for future directions for the study of ADL.

Introduction

Alzheimer's disease (AD) is a debilitating neurodegenerative disease which commonly occurs later in life. Defining characteristics of this disease are memory deficits and other cognitive impairments which infringe upon an individual's ability to live their life normally. In the early stages of AD, everyday tasks such as making a cup of coffee, managing finances and other tasks which require complex interaction with the environment, become difficult for an individual to perform (Rusted & Sheppard, 2002; Tam, Lam, Chiu., & Lui, 2007). These tasks facilitate independent living and quality of life, and are referred to as Instrumental Activities of Daily Living (IADL). However, as this disease progresses, even Basic Activities of Daily Living (BADL), such as bathing, toileting and eating meals, which are fundamental to self-care, become difficult to carry out unaided (Beck & Frank, 1997; Millan-Calenti et al., 2012). Given the large number of people that are living with AD, and as this number is expected to increase over the coming years (Alzheimer's Society, 2014), researchers have attempted to better understand the cognitive processes which underpin the performance of ADL and the neuropsychological tasks which can be used to assess these processes. Such an understanding would allow for better assessment of an individual's functional ability – their ability to independently carry out the daily activities required to meet their basic needs and maintain their health, quality of life and well-being (Manandhar, 1995) – and would facilitate interventions which aim to assist individuals with severe difficulties in maintaining their functional status. This chapter will first discuss the methods that can be used to measure ADL. It will then provide a general overview of the empirical evidence within this research field, which relates to the roles that a range of cognitive abilities provide in performing everyday tasks. Evidence pertaining to the assessment of general cognitive functioning, memory, executive functions, and visuospatial abilities will be explored and issues of ADL and neuropsychological measurement will be discussed. Finally, the neuroimaging portion of this selective review will provide readers with a detailed account of the brain regions thought to underpin ADL performance.

Measuring Activities of Daily Living

Although a subject of much scrutiny by researchers worldwide for some time, no gold standard has yet been set for the measurement of either basic or instrumental ADL. The variety of measurement techniques used by researchers presents an issue for furthering knowledge about which cognitive abilities or brain regions correlate with ADL since certain measurement techniques may be superior to others in assessing ADL accurately, or various measures may assess different aspects of these activities. Thus, it is pertinent that the characteristics of these varying measurement techniques are taken into account when considering the cognitive correlates of ADL.

The four most commonly implemented methods for measuring ADL are:

- Self-report measures.
- Informant-report measures.
- Performance-based measures.
- Direct observation.

Self-Report and Informant-Report Measures of ADL

As with many other psychological phenomena, questionnaire measures present a viable method of measuring ADL. It is common practice for empirical studies to administer self-report measures to healthy individuals, whilst informants such as relatives or professional caregivers are relied upon to provide accounts of cognitively impaired participants' ADL performance. Perhaps one of the most commonly implemented questionnaires for ADL measurement is the Instrumental Activities of Daily Living & Physical Self-Maintenance Scale (IADL-PMS; Lawton & Brody, 1969). This informant-based measure consists of two questionnaires which assess IADL and BADL respectively and comparative norms are widely available. Whilst many researchers have chosen to move on from traditional questionnaire measures to more recently developed techniques, questionnaires such as this one are still widely used for their ease of administration, reproducibility, and due to the fact that these measures are often well-received by participants (Myers, Holliday, Harvey., & Hutchinson, 1993).

Performance-Based Measures of ADL

Despite the apparent benefits of using questionnaire methods to measure ADL, many researchers are reluctant to rely solely upon this method due to the common problem of reporter bias; whilst reports may be accurate in many cases, memory accessibility, attitudes and other internal factors can influence an individual's perception of their own ability or of the ability of a relative/client (Schmitter-Edgecombe, Parsey., & Cook, 2011). Beyond self- and informant- report measures, the development of new measurement techniques has primarily favoured IADL rather than BADL. Impairments of IADL are more subtle, with difficulties in BADL being blatant enough for informant-reports by family members and caregivers to be considered reasonably accurate; difficulties in bathing, walking, toileting, etc., are both easily remembered and easily verified by researchers. Problems in IADL, on the other hand, are less noticeable both to informants and perhaps also to individuals reporting on their own behaviour. Thus, additional techniques have been developed for the assessment of IADL that do not rely upon report measures. One such technique which allows reproduction and standardisation to occur with relative ease is performance-based measures of IADL.

Performance-based measures most commonly come in the form of behavioural simulation tasks, which require participants to perform everyday activities in a laboratory setting. The Multi-Level Action Test (MLAT; Schwartz et al., 1999; Schwartz et al., 1998), for example, requires participants to carry out three tasks under laboratory conditions: making a slice of toast with butter and jam; wrapping a present; and packing a lunchbox. These tasks are repeated several times with various distractions, item-searching or divided-attention conditions present. Behaviour is then coded for overall performance and the types of errors made. Similarly, the Naturalistic Action Test (NAT; Schwartz, Buxbaum, Ferraro, Veramonti., & Segal, 2002) requires participants to carry out these tasks once, with the various conditions being spread out across the three tasks. More recently, behavioural simulation tasks like these have been developed on virtual reality platforms (Allain et al., 2014). Less commonly, performance-based tasks can also come in the form of pen-and-paper tasks which assess the participant's ability to solve real-world challenges. The Everyday Problems Test (EPT; Willis & Marsiske, 1993), for example, assesses the participant's ability to solve problems in seven different IADL domains (meal preparation, medication use, telephone use, shopping, financial management, household management and transportation) using printed materials. For example, a participant might be asked to use drug labels to determine how long a supply of medication will last.

Perhaps the most useful benefit of performance-based measures over questionnaires is that they not only inform researchers about participants' abilities to carry out everyday tasks, they also allow for the types of errors that participants make to be observed and categorised. Several kinds of errors can be consistently observed when individuals carry out everyday tasks and the occurrence of these errors can be informative:

- Irrelevant actions: behaviours which are unnecessary and unrelated to the task.
- Errors of omission: when participants do not complete a particular step of a task.
- Commission errors: when a step in a task is misperformed or an additional step is added.

More specifically, this type of error is comprised of:

- Substitution errors: when alternative, but not correct, objects or actions are used to complete a task.
- Inefficient actions: behaviours which slow the completion of an everyday task.

Although insight into the errors that individuals make can be useful, as will be discussed, performance-based measures have not gone without criticism. It has been argued that these measures are too rigorously controlled to truly reflect everyday behaviour. For example, Myers et al. (1993) maintained that variances in footwear, building structure (stairs, surface types, etc.), and the presence of compensatory tools such as handrails and other environmental adaptations may affect older adults' ADL performance, but performance-based measures are controlled in such a way as to ignore these factors in favour of providing strictly comparable experimental tasks. Additionally, it has been suggested that this strict standardisation can make these tasks difficult to implement (Schmitter-Edgecombe et al., 2011). As a result, more direct measures of ADL performance have been encouraged in recent years.

Direct Observation

Direct observation of a participant's natural behaviour is often encouraged within psychological research, but is also often difficult to implement. Observation of everyday tasks should ideally be done on multiple occasions in the participant's own home. However, funding and recruitment issues often make this impractical. A more accessible substitute for this has been developed, in which observation is done in a pre-prepared naturalistic setting. For example, Schmitter-Edgecombe and Parsey (2014) had participants carry out eight everyday tasks such as watching a DVD and sweeping a floor in a student apartment on campus. This allowed for direct observation to be carried out in a more naturalistic setting than laboratory situated performance-based tasks, whilst still allowing for the coding of task errors. Schmitter-Edgecombe and colleagues have demonstrated using their student apartment observation task that direct observation measures are able to sensitively differentiate between younger adults, older adults of varying ages, cognitively impaired older adults and dementia patients (types unspecified), where report measures and both paper-and-pen and behavioural simulation performance-based measures were less sensitive (Schmitter-Edgecombe et al., 2011; Schmitter-Edgecombe & Parsey, 2014). Based on these findings, these researchers recommend that direct observation be investigated more frequently in future studies, and that this method of measuring ADL may provide a valuable insight into older adults' performance of ADL.

Associations between Cognitive Function and ADL

Global Cognitive Functioning and ADL

In an attempt to understand the cognitive correlates of ADL, researchers have investigated a range of cognitive abilities, including memory, executive functions and visuospatial abilities. A prominent theory in this field, however, is the resource theory of naturalistic action. This theory posits that problems in

ADL result not from specific deficits in any particular cognitive ability, but rather as a result of the overall decline of global cognitive functioning (GCF; Buxbaum, 1998; Schwartz et al., 1999). In support of this theory, Giovannetti, Libon, Buxbaum, and Schwartz (2002) found that GCF, measured using the Mini-Mental State Examination (MMSE), was the strongest predictor of performance (in 51 patients with unspecified dementia) on a short form of the MLAT when compared with measures of executive function (EF) and semantic knowledge. Furthermore, the errors that these dementia patients made on this task were similar to those made by different patient groups (e.g., with closed head injury (Schwartz et al., 1998) or stroke (Schwartz et al., 1999)). With regard to AD specifically, Jefferson, Barakat, Giovannetti, Paul, and Glosser (2006) found that the scores of patients with AD on the MMSE accounted for a significant amount of the variance in their IADL, BADL and total ADL scores, measured using the IADL-PMS (Lawton & Brody, 1969). Based on findings such as these, it has been suggested that GCF is a robust predictor of functional ability in clinical groups.

Although studies such as those above provide evidence to support resource theory, this theory has not gone without challenge. Giovannetti, Schwartz, and Buxbaum (2007) had healthy middle-aged adults carry out a complex coffee task in order to investigate resource limitation in a non-clinical group. They assessed participants' performance of this task when the task was novel to them and when they had practiced the task several times. When the task was well-practiced, they also had participants carry out another simple task at the same time in order to divide the participants' attention and increase the need for cognitive resources. Under these conditions, resource theory would predict a drop in ADL performance due to the increased cognitive demand. What was found, however, was that practising the task repeatedly was enough to maintain good performance of the task even when attention was divided. Giovannetti et al. (2007) suggested that limited resources, then, may not fully account for problems in carrying out ADL. Other studies, such as that by Mioshi, Hodges, and Hornberger (2013) also provide evidence against the theory, finding no significant correlations between GCF (assessed using the Addenbrooke's Cognitive Examination Revised; Mioshi, Dawson, Mitchell, Arnold., & Hodges, 2006) and either IADL or BADL in patients with AD and in patients with fronto-temporal dementia (FTD).

Although GCF may not fully account for ADL problems, this aspect of cognition may still play an influential role in performing everyday tasks through the types of errors that individuals typically perform when carrying out these tasks. For example, Bailey, Kurby, Giovannetti, and Zacks (2013) found in a study of healthy older adults, MCI patients and AD patients that GCF was related to both total performance on the NAT and the amount of Commission errors that occurred. Similarly, GFC was related to AD patients' omissions on the NAT in a study by Giovannetti, Bettcher, Brennan, Libron, et al. (2008). Allain et al. (2014) also demonstrated that AD patients' omissions were associated with GCF in both a virtual reality coffee making simulation and in a real world performance based equivalent. Although studies such as that conducted by Jefferson et al. (2006) highlight the role of GCF in ADL problems in AD patients, their use of report measures prevented an analysis of the types of errors AD patients perform which may relate to GCF. Studies like those above, which examine action errors using performance-based tasks, remedy this problem and provide evidence to support the claim that GCF may not provide an exhaustive account of ADL problems in AD, but can still partially explain these problems through increased errors of omission. Despite this support for the role of GCF in causing omission errors, three of four of the above studies made use of the MMSE (Allain et al., 2014; Giovannetti, Bettcher, Brennan, Libron, et al., 2008; Jefferson et al., 2006), whilst one administered the Clinical Dementia Rating Scale (CDR; Bailey et al., 2013). It is important that more studies test the link between omissions and GCF using tests other than the MMSE. This would confirm whether the results are a product of using this particular test, which focuses primarily on verbal memory.

Memory and ADL

Whilst AD is characterised by a decline in many cognitive abilities, memory impairment is often the most prominent symptom. As such, this cognitive ability has been investigated as a potential factor which underlies the performance of everyday tasks. Evidence relating specifically to AD has been somewhat mixed, with some researchers linking ADL performance to episodic memory (Giovannetti, Bettcher, Brennan, Libron, et al., 2008), whilst others stress the role of semantic memory (Bailey et al., 2013). Semantic memory can be defined as knowledge of facts, words, objects and meaning that is not time-dependent, whilst episodic memory is memory for personal experiences which occurred in particular times and places (Tulving, 1983). Episodic memory impairment is widely regarded as one of the first perceptible symptoms of AD, and as such has been widely investigated with regards to ADL. For example, Giovannetti, Schmidt, Gallo, Sestito, and Libon (2006) carried out a study in which the NAT was administered to AD patients and patients with vascular dementia (VaD). It was found that problems in episodic memory, measured using the Philadelphia repeatable Verbal Learning Test (PVLT; Libon et al., 2005), were associated with problems in everyday functioning in AD patients, but not in VaD patients. This finding emphasises the role of episodic memory in affecting ADL performance in people with AD.

The above studies investigated overall ADL, rather than specific action errors, including errors of omission. In assessing these in 70 AD patients using the NAT, Giovannetti, Bettcher, Brennan, Libron, et al. (2008) noted that episodic memory, measured using the PVLT, was influential in predicting errors of omission. Despite this, Giovannetti, Bettcher, Brennan, Libron, et al. (2008) encouraged caution in interpreting this result as correlations between omission errors and episodic memory were weak, and GCF predicted these errors much more robustly. It seems, then, that there is insufficient evidence relating specifically to AD to conclude that episodic memory impairment solely determines the occurrence of omissions in ADL problems in this disease. It may be the case that episodic memory provides a small contribution to the occurrence of these errors, but further investigation is required. It may also be the case that episodic memory is more closely linked to some other aspect of ADL, such as specific types of everyday tasks. Farias, Harrell, Neumann, and Houtz (2003) used the DAFS and the IADL scale (but not the PMS scale) to assess ADL in AD patients and found that both immediate and delayed episodic memory were significantly related to participant's ability to remember the locations of items. Therefore, it may be that episodic memory, rather than being related to the types of errors described above that AD patients may perform, is related to other difficulties such as locating items which are required to carry out specific tasks. Schmitter-Edgecombe and Parsey (2014) found episodic memory in patients with dementia (types unspecified) and MCI to be more closely linked to IADLs than BADLs, and especially those IADLs which require a greater amount of cognitive processing. These links between episodic memory and impairment on specific types of ADLs should be explored in future research studies. Additional research is also needed to assess the links between ADL and short term and working memory and measures of visual episodic memory, as research to date has primarily focused on verbal episodic memory.

Semantic memory has also been proposed to play a part in the difficulties patients with AD have in performing ADL. Although episodic memory impairments are amongst the first symptoms in AD, semantic memory impairments also occur in most cases (Hodges & Patterson, 1995; Vogel,

Gade, Stokholm, & Waldemar, 2005) and so it comes as no surprise that this cognitive sub-domain has been investigated with regards to ADL in AD. More general research into ADL and clinical groups has proposed that semantic memory problems affect ADL performance through poor representations of tasks and the objects needed to perform these, which potentially causes an increase in omissions (Hartmann, Goldenberg, Daumüller, & Hermsdörfer, 2005; Ochipa, Rothi, & Heilman, 1989). Bailey et al. (2013) aimed to investigate this further in order to determine if an individual's ability to mentally represent events which typically occur in everyday life is related to their performance of everyday tasks. They assessed participants' ability to mentally represent events by having them observe movie clips of typical events, such as a woman checking a book out of a library, and segment these clips into sequences of meaningful actions by pressing the space bar every time the actor completed a meaningful action in the event. In the library example, participants might be expected to press the space bar when the actor selected a book, approached the reception desk, engaged with the librarian, handed over their library card, etc. Whilst traditional tests of semantic memory (animal naming, Boston Naming Task and the WAIS information subtest) were not significantly related to performance on the NAT and omission errors, participants' ability to segment events were. Therefore, it is possible that event models, which can draw upon relevant information from both episodic and semantic memory, are related to the ability to carry out everyday tasks in AD. This is consistent with the fact that several other studies have assessed ADL in AD patients using traditional tests of semantic memory (the Boston Naming Test and Pyramids and Palm Trees, respectively) and found no relationship (Giovannetti, Bettcher, Brennan, Libron, et al., 2008; Jefferson et al., 2006). Studies of this kind, however, are infrequent and so, whilst it seems that Bailey et al. (2013) have made progress in clarifying how semantic knowledge might be related to the performance of everyday tasks in AD, more research is required which assess the events model of AD patients. Further to this, much work is required in order to determine which method of measuring these representations ought to be considered most appropriate for this undertaking.

Executive Functions and ADL

Given the role of executive functions (EF), such as reasoning, planning and problem solving, in facilitating the performance of complicated, goal-directed behaviours (Bell-McGinty, Podell, Franzen, Baird, & Williams,

2002), an association between this subset of cognitive abilities and ADL function might be expected. In support of this notion, a variety of studies have found EF to be a significant predictor of ADL performance in healthy older adults (Bell-McGinty et al., 2002; Cahn-Weiner, Malloy, Boyle, Marran, & Salloway, 2000; Grigsby, Kaye, Baxter, Shetterly, & Hamman, 1998; Lewis & Miller, 2007), and in patients with vascular dementia (Giovannetti et al., 2006). Furthermore, case studies of patients with executive control impairments (Buxbaum, Schwartz, & Carew, 1997) and problems in goal-directed behaviour (Duncan, 1986) have linked EF to ADL performance. In the study on dementia patients conducted by Schmitter-Edgecombe and Parsey (2014), EF showed prominence in affecting functional ability; EF was found to be related to inefficient actions, a sub-group of errors which are related to commissions. Bell-McGinty et al. (2002) aimed to assess the usefulness of a variety of standardised measures of EF which are commonly used in clinical settings using healthy older adults and found that the Trail Making Test – Part B and the Wisconsin Card Sorting Test (WCST-64) were the best predictors of ADL performance.

Several studies have focused on the role of EF in AD patients' performance of ADL. Although these have found EF to be generally associated with ADL (e.g., Cahn-Weiner et al., 2007; Cahn-Weiner, Ready, & Malloy, 2003; Chen, Sultzer, Hinkin, Mahler, & Cummings, 1998; Marshall et al., 2011; see also the recent meta-analysis by Martyr & Clare, 2012), a growing number of studies have investigated the relationship between EF and ADL with specific regard to action errors. This research has consistently demonstrated a link between EF and commission errors. Allain et al. (2014) used the non-immersive virtual coffee task (NI-VCT) and a performance-based task to demonstrate a link between EF and commission errors in AD patients. Similarly, commission errors performed by AD patients during the NAT have been linked to EF (Bailey et al., 2013; Giovannetti, Bettcher, Brennan, Libron, et al., 2008). In the study by Farias et al. (2003), EF predicted AD patients' ability to write a check and balance a chequebook as part of the DAFS, and shop, measured by Lawton's IADL. As a result of these studies, there is evidence to suggest that executive control underpins the occurrence of commission errors in ADL performance in AD, and that this cognitive ability might be drawn upon to perform financially-based ADL. Despite this, few studies have investigated which tests of EF might predict these impairments most informatively. Allain et al. (2014) opted to test EF using the Frontal Assessment Battery (FAB; Dubois, Slachevsky, Litvan, & Pillon, 2000), whilst Farias et al. (2003) chose to assess this cognitive domain using the Controlled Oral Word Association (COWA) test (Benton & de Hamsher, 1989) and the Similarities subtest of the Wechsler Adults Intelligence Test – Revised (Wechsler, 1981), and both Giovannetti, Bettcher, Brennan, Libron, et al. (2008) and Bailey et al. (2013) used the revised and original version of the WMS Mental Control sub-test (Wechsler, 1945), respectively. It is entirely possible that EF predicts commission errors in AD so robustly that any measure of EF which taps this cognitive ability with relative precision would be appropriate for use in this kind of research. However, it would be valuable for future studies to comparatively investigate various EF tasks, as Bell-McGinty et al. (2002) did, but with regard to AD patients and the commission errors that they perform. Such a study may reveal the superiority of one or more EF tasks in linking executive control to ADL performance in AD patients.

Visuospatial Abilities and ADL

A final cognitive correlate of ADL that this chapter will explore is visuospatial abilities. Visuospatial impairment is a lesser known symptom of AD, which typically becomes evident in the mid-to-late stages of this disease (Frisoni et al., 2008; McDonald et al., 2009). In an attempt to understand the role of this impairment in ADL performance, Fukui & Lee (2009) had 57 AD patients carry out the IADL-PMS. They found that visuo-construction, measured using the Clock Drawing Test (CDT) predicted difficulties in BADL, and that visuo-perception, measured using the Clock Reading Test (CRT), was related to both BADL difficulty and IADL difficulty. Similarly, it was found by Jefferson et al. (2006) that AD patients' performance of BADL and IADL based on the IADL-PMS was predicted by object perception. In a study of Spanish and English AD patients, Loewenstein, Rubert, Arguelles, and Duara (1995) also found visuospatial ability, measured using the Block Design task, to be related to ADL performance, this time using the DAFS. In a more in depth investigation of IADLs, both Farias et al. (2003) and Glosser et al. (2002) found visuospatial ability to be linked to specific types of everyday tasks; Farias et al. (2003) found this cognitive domain to be linked to the ability to write a cheque and address a letter, whilst Glosser et al. (2002) found an association between visuospatial abilities and other visually based IADLs, such as driving and recognising people. Several studies have investigated visuospatial abilities and have found no relationships between this cognitive ability and ADL performance (Giovannetti, Bettcher, Brennan, Libron, et al.,

2008; Schmitter-Edgecombe & Parsey, 2014). However, these studies have either not looked specifically at AD (Schmitter-Edgecombe & Parsey, 2014), or have investigated categories of action errors rather than categories of ADL, such as visually-based tasks (Giovannetti, Bettcher, Brennan, Libon, et al., 2008). Since visuospatial ability is affected through the course of AD (Frisoni et al., 2008; McDonald et al., 2009) and the above studies have found impaired visuospatial abilities to be related to the performance of visually-based activities in AD patients (Farias et al., 2003; Glosser et al., 2002), it is reasonable to conclude that visuospatial ability does impact upon AD patients' ability to carry out everyday tasks, if these tasks are visually based. However, the studies which support this conclusion have used a variety of different visuospatial measures. Comparing various visuospatial measures and how they link to ADLs could be beneficial in guiding ADL interventions and in determining the difficulties that patients with AD face in completing different kinds of everyday tasks.

Summary: Cognitive Correlates of ADL

Investigation of the cognitive correlates of ADL has been an ongoing pursuit for several decades. A small portion of this research is dedicated specifically to the investigation of AD patients' performance of everyday tasks and an exploration of this research has revealed several cognitive correlates of AD patients' functional ability. Additionally, it has highlighted the variety of neuropsychological tasks which have been used to investigate these domains. With regard to GCF, research to date has suggested that a primary route through which GCF explains ADL performance, in patients with AD is through the production of omission errors when carrying out everyday tasks. Much of this research, however, has made use of the MMSE when assessing AD patients. As a result, it would be prudent for future research to investigate the relationship between AD patients' omission errors using alternative tests of GCF, in order to ensure that this finding is not the product of a particular test.

Unlike GCF, evidence pertaining to the influence of episodic memory in AD and ADL has produced rather unclear findings. There is currently insufficient evidence to clarify the role of episodic memory in either general ADL performance or in the production of omission errors. Research which assesses episodic memory using a variety of tests, both verbal and visual, is required. This should ideally be done using an investigation of different domains of IADL, BADL and of the types of action errors that AD patients perform. As for the role of semantic memory in ADL, much of research in this field has investigated this using traditional tests of semantic knowledge and language and has found no significant relationships in AD patients (Bailey et al., 2013; Giovannetti, Bettcher, Brennan, Libron, et al., 2008; Jefferson et al., 2006).

However, preliminary research suggests that this may be because semantic memory influences ADL performance in AD patients' through their representation of events (Bailey et al., 2013). More research is required on this topic in order to conclusively determine if this is the case or not, but this remains a promising avenue for future studies.

Whilst research into event modelling has been quite sparse, research investigating the role of EF in AD patients' performance of everyday tasks has conversely been quite extensive, and there is strong evidence to support the claim that problems in EF are associated with both general ADL function and the occurrence of commission errors in AD. These investigations have used a variety of neuropsychological tasks, and future research could conduct research studies to compare the contribution of these various measures of EF to ADL.

As for the study of visuospatial abilities, research suggests that, rather than being linked to overall ADL performance, or any particular type of error made by AD patients, visuospatial abilities are linked to specific kinds of ADL; namely ADL which are visually-based and so require increased visuospatial processing. As with the other cognitive domains, it is important that comparative studies of different visuospatial tasks are carried out in order to clarify their relationship to ADL.

Functional Neuroimaging of ADL

The literature that has attempted to isolate the brain regions that are associated with ADL impairment will now be explored. The following set of studies used either Single Photon Emission Computed Tomography (SPECT) or Positron Emission Tomography (PET) to assess regional brain perfusion/metabolism respectively.

Associations between Regional Brain Perfusion/Metabolism and ADL

Using Lawton's IADL scale, Salmon et al. (2005) demonstrated in a large sample of patients with probable AD, and using a whole-brain voxel-based analysis, that IADL was associated with lower metabolism in the right temporoparietal cortex and the left superior occipital gyrus. Melrose and colleagues (2011) similarly showed, in a group of patients with AD, that lower functionality in everyday abilities (again assessed with the Lawton IADL scale) was associated with hypometabolism across a set of right sided regions - the temporoparietal cortex, dorsolateral prefrontal cortex (DLPFC), frontal pole, and thalamus. Path analysis involving three regions of interest (ROIs) centred on the right DLPFC, frontal pole and inferior parietal lobule revealed that the metabolic associations with IADL tended to be attenuated when the MMSE was included in a multiple regression model, which suggests that GCF partly mediates the relationship (Melrose et al., 2011). Given that performance on the MMSE did not fully eliminate the relationships with all ROIs, and that the behavioural studies described above demonstrated numerous links between specific cognitive functions and ADL (general performance and errors), the combination of a variety of tests measuring cognitive functions such as EF, visuospatial abilities, and episodic memory, might be an even stronger mediator of the relationship between brain metabolism and IADL abilities.

Impairment in driving ability in patients with AD, as reported by caregivers, has also been linked to temporoparietal (and occipital) hypoperfusion, possibly indicating visuospatial/perceptual difficulties (a conclusion supported by the finding of an association with the CDT – copy requirement) (Ott et al., 2000). More severe impairment which prevented driving altogether on the other hand was associated with frontal hypoperfusion, possibly relating to difficulties with EFs that occur later in the disease course (Ott et al., 1996). This hypothesis was supported by the finding of an association with clock drawing (both in copying and drawing to command). The ability to drive was also strongly associated with IADL (assessed with Lawton's IADL scale).

It seems that across these studies one of the consistent findings in patients with AD, is that reduced perfusion/metabolism within or in the proximity of the right temporoparietal cortex is associated with impairment in IADL functioning. Melrose et al. (2011) highlighted that this might relate to the visual nature of IADLs (e.g., shopping, housecleaning). The parietal cortex is a component of the dorsal processing stream, which is associated with the representation of objects in space and visually guided movement, whereas the temporal cortex is a part of the ventral processing stream, which is linked to object recognition. Right-sided brain regions, such as the parietal cortex, also underpin processes such as visual working memory and play a major role in attentional processing (Melrose et al., 2011). The brain regions listed above additionally comprise elements of the dorsal and ventral attentional networks (Corbetta, Patel, & Shulman, 2008), which together provide top-down control, the ability to reorient attention, select stimuli for processing and link these to responses - functions that would be expected to be important for successful IADL performance.

Associations between Brain Perfusion and Discrete Components of ADL

A recent SPECT study by Nadkarni et al. (2012) contributed further to the literature, by dividing the scores on the Disability Assessment for Dementia (DAD) (Gelinas, Gauthier, McIntyre, & Gauthier, 1999) into an ADL initiation score, and ADL planning/preparation score and an ADL execution/performance score. Correlations between the total ADL score and each of these separate scores were assessed against perfusion across a set of ROIs. Total ADL correlated positively with perfusion in the right superior parietal ROI. This finding fits well with the earlier studies that were described above (Melrose et al., 2011; Ott et al., 2000; Salmon et al., 2005) and as mentioned, the right parietal cortex may be important for functions such as spatial attention, motor planning, and visuospatial integration (Nadkarni et al., 2012). Total ADL score also correlated negatively with depression score (recorded via the Cornell Depression Scale). The nature of such a relationship may relate to depression caused by lower ADL ability, or depression may arise contemporaneously with ADL impairment due to pathological involvement of the brain regions that underpin both. For example, higher levels of depression have been shown to be associated with hypometabolism within the parietal cortex (e.g., Sultzer et al., 1995).

Splitting the ADL measure into its components showed that ADL planning/preparation correlated with perfusion within the right occipital ROI, and ADL execution/performance with the right superior parietal ROI. ADL Initiation was associated with perfusion within ROIs in the right frontal pole and in the DLPFC, VLPFC, ACC and caudate/putamen bilaterally. The relationship between initiation and the fronto-striatal circuits may reflect impairment to executive functions (e.g., initiation and decision making) (Nadkarni et al., 2012). The link between ADL initiation and the PFC, ACC and striatum also fits well with findings that show associations between these brain regions and apathy (Bruen, McGeown, Shanks, & Venneri, 2008; Lanctot et al., 2007; Marshall et al., 2007; Migneco et al., 2001). Furthermore, the striatum is involved in motor control and the shifting of spatial attention, in addition to learning (during tasks where response strategies must be selected), which highlights the contribution these subcortical nuclei may make to procedural knowledge (a memory system likely to strongly underpin ADLs) (Brown, Schneider, & Lidsky, 1997; Mesulam, 2000; Phillips & Carr, 1987).

Regional Brain Perfusion/Metabolism to Predict Decline in ADL

Neuroimaging studies have also investigated whether the level of perfusion/metabolism within certain regions of the brain can predict future decline in ADL. Being able to more accurately predict future impairment could enable more informed planning in relation to the level of assistance that will be required, and might assist the design of effective interventions. An early study by Nobili et al. (2001) assessed the relationship between regional cerebral blood flow (rCBF) and BADL (eating, bathing, dressing) in patients with AD. An analysis restricted to a posterior temporal/inferior parietal ROI in each hemisphere revealed that rCBF within both ROIs predicted future decline. Furthermore, the relationship was maintained when a multiple regression model was created, with MMSE, age, age of onset, disease duration, sex, and the presence of psychotic symptoms and extrapyramidal symptoms entered as covariates. Similarly, a more recent study by Landau et al. (2011) on patients with AD and MCI showed that lower levels of metabolism measured within a composite ROI, that included the temporoparietal cortex, and posterior cingulate bilaterally, predicted future declines in functionality on ADL (as measured with the Functional Activities Questionnaire). A limitation of these studies was that the entire cortex was not assessed for predictive power and it may be that other brain regions (or combinations of brain regions) would make even better predictors.

In sum, metabolism/perfusion within the temporoparietal cortex measured at baseline can predict ADL decline over time. Interestingly, in the study by Landau et al. (2011), a further finding (in the patients with AD) was that the metabolic measurement offered more predictive power than a cognitive screening scale – the ADAS-cog. This suggests that these types of functional neuroimaging measures, if refined and validated further, could be utilized for more accurate prognosis in the future. The study did not assess the utility of specific neuropsychological tests in comparison to the metabolic measures in predicting ADL decline however.

Summary: Functional Neuroimaging of ADL

In summary, an evidence base is accumulating that links decreased performance in ADLs in patients with AD to the temporoparietal cortex, especially within the right hemisphere (Melrose et al., 2011; Nadkarni et al., 2012; Ott et al., 2000; Salmon et al., 2005). The studies have also demonstrated potential links to a more extensive set of brain regions, which has included bilateral regions of the VLPFC, DLPFC, ACC, striatum and occipital cortex, and the right frontal pole and thalamus (Melrose et al., 2011; Nadkarni et al., 2012; Ott et al., 2000; Salmon et al., 2005). As mentioned above, the right temporoparietal cortex has a number of roles that once impaired could affect ADL function. These regions of the cortex relate to attentional processing, visuomotor integration, motor planning and working memory (Nadkarni et al., 2012). The temporoparietal (and occipital cortex) are also related to visuospatial/perceptual processes, and evidence exists which links such processes to ADL performance (Farias et al., 2003; Fukui & Lee, 2009; Glosser et al., 2002; Hill, Backman, & Fratiglioni, 1995; Jefferson et al., 2006; Mahurin, DeBettignies, & Pirozzolo, 1991). That the associations between ADLs involve mostly right lateralized brain regions might have particular significance. As Melrose et al., (2011) highlight, IADLs generally require visual processing and environmental interaction, and the right hemisphere is particularly involved in planning movements, visual working memory and in attentional control processes.

Frontal involvement was associated with an inability to drive, but not estimates of less severe impairment which were instead linked more closely to visuospatial processing. Although driving estimations correlated with IADLs, driving itself could be classed as an IADL. If the frontal involvement predominantly reflects executive dysfunction, this might signify that a critical threshold is being crossed, and that once the disease progresses beyond this stage, patients will not be able to rely on EFs for the performance of the ADL tasks. Furthermore if EFs are viewed as a resource that may help to compensate for other impairments, their depletion would have an additional and marked impact on the performance of everyday tasks. The progression of brain hypometabolism/perfusion from the temporoparietal to frontal brain regions fits with the natural progression of AD (see e.g., Herholz et al., 2002; Minoshima et al., 1997) and the behavioural literature on ADLs has demonstrated links between EFs and everyday functioning (Bell-McGinty et al., 2002; Cahn-Weiner, Boyle, & Malloy, 2002; Grigsby et al., 1998; Lewis & Miller, 2007). Further to this, fronto-striatal dysfunction associated with ADL impairment, might relate to difficulties with executive processing, procedural knowledge, and motor control.

Structural Neuroimaging of ADL

The studies that have employed structural neuroimaging methods to investigate ADL will now be reviewed. In the same fashion that ADL scores can be correlated with perfusion and/or metabolic measures, associations can also be explored between ADL scores and structural measures such as grey matter (GM) volume.

Associations between Neuroanatomical Measures and ADL in AD

Cahn-Weiner et al. (2007) assessed whether neuropsychological and/or structural neuroimaging measures were associated with baseline IADL and whether they could predict future IADL decline. The Blessed Roth Dementia Rating Scale (Blessed, Tomlinson, & Roth, 1988) provided the measure of IADL across a heterogeneous sample of 24 patients with possible/probable AD, 7 with possible/probable ischemic VaD, 6 with mixed dementia (AD/cerebrovascular disease), 35 with MCI, and 52 controls. Individual models showed that composite scores for memory and EF, total cortical GM and hippocampal volume (HV) were associated with IADL baseline scores and predicted future decline. To assess the independent contribution of each of the different data types, a joint model was also created which included the neuropsychological and neuroimaging data. Memory and HV were independently associated with baseline IADL. EF, however, emerged as the only predictor of IADL change. This finding further supports the idea described in the previous section that decline in EF might signify a critical boundary, in which additional impairment to these functions will severely impact ADL functionality. It also flags the potential utility of measuring EFs for prognostic purposes. A further finding in the study, relating to the demographics, was that higher education at baseline was independently associated with better performance in IADLs (while covarying for age, memory and EF). Education was also associated with IADL change over time (while accounting for variance associated with age, GM and HV). It seems that higher levels of education may protect patients from ADL decline; a finding that resonates with some other research findings (e.g., Marshall et al., 2011).

Using whole-brain voxel-based morphometry (VBM) on patients with AD, Vidoni et al. (2010) examined which brain regions were associated with lower levels of cognition, physical function and ADL ability (using the Alzheimer's Disease Cooperative Study-Activities of Daily Living Scale; ADCS-ADL) in patients with AD. A global conjunction analysis showed that the independent variables were associated with GM volume within the right temporoparietal cortex, hippocampus, and parahippocampus, and within the left inferior and superior frontal gyri. In line with these findings, and also using VBM, but with the added advantage of utilizing the DAD, which can provide separate IADL and BADL scores (in addition to a total score), Mioshi et al., (2013) showed that BADL performance was mostly associated with the temporoparietal regions, in addition to, for example, the PFC, cingulate cortex, caudate, hippocampus and parahippocampus. The more complex and demanding IADLs were associated with a reasonably similar, but more extensive pattern of regional involvement that also incorporated the right lateral occipital cortex. As in the functional neuroimaging studies, associations between ADL and the temporoparietal cortices were detected across these structural neuroimaging studies, however unlike the former, the majority of which were restricted to ROI analyses (and excluded examination of the MTL), the two structural neuroimaging studies that adopted whole-brain voxel-wise analyses, flagged associations between the hippocampus and parahippocampus, and ADL. These associations appear to complement the behavioural findings that relate episodic memory to ADL function (e.g., Farias et al., 2003; Giovannetti et al., 2006).

In summary, similar to the functional neuroimaging studies, this set of neuroanatomical studies showed that ADL function is associated with GM volume within the temporoparietal cortex, in addition to the PFC and cingulate cortex. Additional relationships were also revealed, however, between ADL and the hippocampus/parahippocampus (Cahn-Weiner et al., 2007; Mioshi et al., 2013; Vidoni et al., 2010). The results also show that IADL and BADL appear to rely on similar brain regions. As may be expected, the more complex

IADLs were associated with a more diverse set of brain regions, however, and these are likely to underpin a wider variety of cognitive functions.

Associations between Neuroanatomical Measures and ADL in Other Types of Dementia

The relationships between ADL and neuroimaging measures in patients with AD can also be contrasted to those in other types of dementia. In addition to patients with AD, Mioshi et al. (2013) also assessed patients with FTD, finding that better BADL performance was associated with higher GM volume within the left medial frontal cortex, para-cingulate, and the frontal pole, bilaterally. IADLs linked to GM integrity within similar brain regions, but as in the patients with AD, a greater number of brain regions were implicated. More specifically, these included extensive portions of the bilateral PFC, in addition to the left posterior cingulate, and the right thalamus, cerebellum, and hippocampus. Associations were also detected in the occipital poles and lateral occipital cortex, bilaterally. Despite some degree of overlap across patient groups, in FTD the relationship between ADL and regional GM appears to be much more strongly focused on the PFC, whereas in AD the relationship is more widespread and incorporates more posterior regions such as the temporoparietal cortex. We have highlighted above the role of the PFC in executive functions and that these are likely to support ADL function. Such strong associations between the PFC (and ACC) and ADL in patients with FTD are likely to further reflect these functions, but additionally might reflect the behavioural symptoms in FTD and how they may be strong drivers in determining the level of everyday functioning (Mioshi et al., 2007). Only one brain region, the left superior frontal cortex was associated with IADL in both patient groups. This brain region has been linked to task-switching (Cutini et al., 2008), action planning and the control of complex movements (Majdandzic et al., 2007; Martino et al., 2011), and working memory, especially when the demands are complex in nature and in the spatial domain (du Boisgueheneuc et al., 2006).

Chow et al. (2008) further showed that ADL performance in patients with FTD was associated with GM in ROIs that encompassed the striatum and thalamus bilaterally. The study only focused on these subcortical nuclei however and did not explore associations between ADL and other brain regions. The potential implications of damage to fronto-striatal circuits in contributing to difficulties in ADL were discussed above. Given the roles of the thalamic regions, in the processing of perceptual information, impairment might be expected to contribute to a breakdown in ADL, as demonstrated in the studies of FTD (Chow et al., 2008; Mioshi et al., 2013) and AD (Salmon et al., 2005). The thalamus has also been linked to apathetic behaviour (Marshall et al., 2007).

Turning now to patients with VaD, Boyle et al., (2003) found that EF explained 28% of the variance in IADLs (Lawton's IADL scale) and WMHs explained a further 14%. These findings contrast with those of Cahn-Weiner et al., (2007), who did not find any association between WMH (or lacunar volume) and baseline IADL or IADL over time. The discrepancy might have arisen due to the differences in the primary neuropathologies in each participant sample (Cahn-Weiner et al., 2007). Cahn-Weiner et al. included a mix of patients (the majority of whom had AD, whereas a lesser number had VaD, and mixed dementia (AD/CVD)), while Boyle et al. had patients with suspected VaD only. The main pathologies in AD take the form of amyloid plaques and neurofibrillary tangles, whereas WMH changes may be less severe until later in the disease course resulting in reduced opportunity to detect associations between the vascular factors and ADL.

Overall, compared to AD, difficulties in ADL in patients with FTD appear to be linked predominantly to anterior regions of the brain. ADLs were associated mostly with the PFC, and with other brain regions including the cingulate cortex, striatum and thalamus. The studies demonstrate that the type of neuropathology and its distribution in each disorder, as one might expect, determines which brain regions are most strongly associated with deficits in ADL, presumably (as the behavioural studies indicate) due to disease-related impairments in multiple cognitive and behavioural functions.

Summary: Structural Neuroimaging of ADL

The structural neuroimaging studies on patients with AD complement the functional neuroimaging findings, showing that ADLs were associated with a set of brain regions which included the temporoparietal cortex, PFC and cingulate cortex. The studies also highlighted further links between ADL and the hippocampus/parahippocampus, however. The associations between ADL function and low hippocampal/parahippocampal volume may partially reflect the relationship between episodic memory and ADL that has been shown in the behavioural literature (Farias et al., 2003; Giovannetti et al., 2006). It should be noted that links between ADL impairment and episodic memory could reflect these problems within the MTLs, but might also be related to the dysfunction of memory processes based within the frontal lobes (e.g., encoding, retrieval processes; Cabeza & Nyberg, 2000).

As discussed above, impairment to the temporoparietal cortex may lead to deficits in attention, visuospatial processing and visual working memory. The relationship between atrophy in the fronto-striatal regions and decreased everyday abilities may well relate to executive dysfunction, an assumption supported by the literature which illustrates links between these brain regions and EFs (e.g., Pa et al., 2010; Ragozzino, 2007; Rowe & Passingham, 2001; Smith & Jonides, 1999), and by behavioural studies which demonstrate associations between EFs and ADLs (Bell-McGinty et al., 2002; Cahn-Weiner et al., 2002; Cahn-Weiner et al., 2000). It should also be noted however, that although some neuropsychological tasks that are used to assess EF are classically thought to be associated with the frontal lobes, such complex tasks require support from many other regions of the cortex. For example the Trail Making Test (Part B) does not appear to be associated only with the frontal lobe (Chan et al., 2015), but also with multiple brain regions which include the right posterior parietal lobe (Pa et al., 2010). In this sense the strong associations between the measures of EF produced with such tasks and ADL, are likely not to be due only to frontal dysfunction, but also to impairment in other brain regions which are associated with ADL performance such as the temporoparietal cortex.

Comparing the results of the ADL studies on patients with AD to those that involved patients with other types of dementia shows that the brain regions that correlate most closely with ADL function, as might be expected, are those that relate most strongly to the distribution of neuropathological features and the pattern of atrophy (and hypoperfusion/metabolism) that occurs in each type of dementia. In this sense, ADLs relate to overall disease severity, and the reports of associations between ADL and measures of GCF (e.g., in the studies of Giovannetti et al., 2002; Jefferson et al., 2006) might be explained in this manner. Additional analyses within the study by Salmon et al. (2005) can illustrate this point. In the same patient group there was overlap in the brain regions that correlated with MMSE score and those that correlated with IADL (e.g., the left PFC, and the temporoparietal cortex, bilaterally). With this in mind, future neuroimaging studies might want to create multiple regression models to examine associations between neuroimaging measures and ADL, while covarying for overall disease severity (with measures such as the MMSE or CDR). This approach might help to identify the brain regions or networks that are most closely related to ADL function. As this approach might of course remove variance that is associated with ADL performance, analyses with and without the inclusion of a measure of GCF should be performed.

Conclusion

This chapter has explored the four commonly used techniques for measuring ADL which have emerged in the research literature over the past few decades. Each of these techniques: self-report, informant-report, performance-based tasks, and direct observation – have relative advantages and disadvantages. Report-measures, whilst being easy to administer and reproduce, are subject to report bias and do not provide information on the types of errors produced by individuals. Performance-based tasks allow for this, but are highly standardised and rigorously controlled and so may have low ecological validity. Direct observation improves upon this validity issue, but this method can be difficult to implement and requires further validation by future research. It is important that the interpretation of research findings be considered in light of the ADL measurement technique used. This is because each of these techniques may have been used to provide valuable insights throughout the ADL literature, but they may do so by shedding light on different aspects of ADL. As such, the role of each of these techniques in informing research ought to be carefully considered in future, and the appropriate technique(s) should be selected depending upon the nature of the study in which they are used, in order to optimise the advantages of these ADL measurement techniques.

The role that GCF, memory, EF and visuospatial abilities play in AD patients' performance of ADL has been discussed. Whilst much of the research into the cognitive correlates of ADL in AD patients requires further clarification and investigation, a general overview of the current research evidence suggests that: GCF likely plays a role in AD patients' performance through general performance of tasks and through the occurrence of errors of omission; the role of episodic memory in ADL is unclear, but this cognitive ability may contribute partially to AD patients' performance of omission errors also; semantic memory may influence the performance of everyday tasks in AD patients through their representations of everyday events; EF likely influences AD patients' functional ability through the occurrence of commission errors; and finally, visuospatial abilities appear to influence everyday task performance when tasks require visual processing. In order to provide further support for these preliminary conclusions, future research must investigate a wider variety of neuropsychological tasks for each of these domains, whilst assessing different domains of IADL and BADL, and using appropriate measures of ADL. This is because research to date has primarily been conducted using only one neuropsychological task per cognitive ability (e.g., MMSE to measure GCF, COWA to measure EF etc.), rather than administering a range of neuropsychological tasks in order to determine which tests are most appropriate for measuring each of these domains of cognition in relation to ADL. Furthermore, few research studies have investigated the cognitive correlates of ADL with regard to the different kinds of IADL that are carried out on a daily basis, and with regard to BADL. As a result, there is considerable room for further clarification of the cognitive correlates of ADL by future research.

The neuroimaging studies on patients with AD, consistently revealed associations between ADL and the temporoparietal cortex. Other brain regions that were linked to ADL included the PFC, the cingulate cortex, the striatum, the hippocampus/parahippocampus and the occipital cortex. These brain regions are known to underpin a variety of cognitive functions, including EFs, visuospatial functions, and episodic/semantic memory. The findings fit well with those of the behavioural studies discussed above which found associations between these cognitive functions and ADL. As AD progresses, increased dysfunction occurs across multiple cognitive domains (which contribute to greater decline in GCF), and consequently there is greater impairment to various ADLs. The level of contribution of the neural dysfunction within different brain regions to ADL impairment is still not overly clear however. Despite this, we can still draw some conclusions given the available data. As individuals with amnestic MCI tend to have deterioration within the MTLs, but tend to display only discreet and subtle problems in certain complex IADLs, this suggests that more marked ADL impairment occurs only once neuropathology and neural dysfunction spreads to other brain regions. In support of this notion, in those people with MCI who also have executive dysfunction in addition to memory difficulties, greater functional difficulties are noted (Marshall et al., 2011). Conversion to dementia also involves progression of the neuropathology to other brain regions, and this appears to be when a marked drop in ADL occurs. Further support is provided by the evidence that demonstrates strong associations between ADL and EF, between ADL and visual-spatial abilities, and between ADL and the frontal and temporo-parietal-occipital neuroimaging measures.

By dividing their patient group on the severity of ADL impairment, Ott et al. (2000) also clearly show a shift towards frontal associations with ADL, when driving impairments becomes so severe that the patient is no longer fit to drive, suggesting that neuropathology has progressed to the PFC at that time. To better inform intervention designs, additional studies are needed to assess which brain regions play the greatest role in ADL problems (and these could covary for disease severity and/or assess the independent contribution and potential mediation of a range of cognitive functions using multiple regression models). Patients could be subdivided by disease stage, the level of ADL impairment, or even by impairment on specific ADL items, to assess the differential contribution of cognitive/neuroimaging measures. Further to this performance-based/direct observation methods should be used to assess ADL, as error analyses in neuroimaging studies appear to be lacking despite the increased popularity of such measures in the behavioural literature.

The results of two studies suggested that functional neuroimaging measures (ROIs in the temporoparietal cortex, and one which included the posterior cingulate cortex) may predict ADL decline (Landau et al., 2011; Nobili et al., 2001). While the results of each of these suggest that the neuroimaging measures provide additional benefits for prognosis, than GCF measures alone, a structural neuroimaging study showed that a specific cognitive measure (EF) was the only significant predictor of ADL decline when the neuroimaging measures of HV and the crude neuroimaging variable of total cortical brain volume were entered in the model (Cahn-Weiner et al., 2007). To assist patient management and the ability of patient's and relatives to plan for the future, a need is evident for additional studies to apply a wider range neuroimaging measures (e.g., further ROIs possibly determined through voxel-based analyses) and more measures of cognition, to determine which assessments (or more likely combination of assessments) offers the most accurate prognosis.

In summary, this chapter has highlighted the different methods that have been and could be used in the study of ADL in patients with AD, it has shown which cognitive functions correlate with ADL performance and ADL error types, and it has highlighted the brain regions that most closely link to performance on everyday tasks. Future studies will expand this growing research area and have the potential to provide insight into which cognitive functions could be assessed as proxy measures for ADL in clinical trials, which content and format personalised interventions should take, and how cognitive/neuroimaging measures may enable more accurate prognosis.

References

Allain, P., Foloppe, D. A., Besnard, J., Yamaguchi, T., Etcharry-Bouyx, F., Le Gall, D., Nolan, P. & Richard, P. (2014). Detecting everyday action deficits in Alzheimer's disease using a nonimmersive virtual reality kitchen. *J Int Neuropsychol Soc*, *20*(5), 468-477. doi: 10.1017/s1355617714000344

Alzheimer's Society. (2014). Demography. Retrieved May 13th, 2015, from http://www.alzheimers.org.uk/site/scripts/documents_info.php?documentID=412

Bailey, H. R., Kurby, C. A., Giovannetti, T. & Zacks, J. M. (2013). Action perception predicts action performance. *Neuropsychologia*, *51*(11), 2294-2304. doi: http://dx.doi.org/10.1016/j.neuropsychologia.2013.06.022

Beck, C. K. & Frank, L. B. (1997). Assessing functioning and self-care abilities in Alzheimer disease research. *Alzheimer Dis Assoc Disord, 11 Suppl 6*, 73-80.

Bell-McGinty, S., Podell, K., Franzen, M., Baird, A. D. & Williams, M. J. (2002). Standard measures of executive function in predicting instrumental activities of daily living in older adults. *Int J Geriatr Psychiatry*, *17*(9), 828-834. doi: 10.1002/gps.646

Benton, A. L. & de Hamsher, K. S. (1989). *Multilingual Aphasia examination.* Iowa City, IA: AJA Associates.

Blessed, G., Tomlinson, B. E. & Roth, M. (1988). Blessed-Roth Dementia Scale (DS). *Psychopharmacol Bull*, *24*(4), 705-708.

Boyle, P. A., Paul, R., Moser, D., Zawacki, T., Gordon, N. & Cohen, R. (2003). Cognitive and neurologic predictors of functional impairment in vascular dementia. *Am J Geriatr Psychiatry*, *11*(1), 103-106.

Brown, L. L., Schneider, J. S. & Lidsky, T. I. (1997). Sensory and cognitive functions of the basal ganglia. *Curr Opin Neurobiol*, *7*(2), 157-163.

Bruen, P. D., McGeown, W. J., Shanks, M. F. & Venneri, A. (2008). Neuroanatomical correlates of neuropsychiatric symptoms in Alzheimer's disease. *Brain*, *131*(Pt 9), 2455-2463.

Buxbaum, L. J. (1998). Ideational apraxia and naturalistic action. *Cogn Neuropsychol*, *15*(6-8), 617-643. doi: 10.1080/026432998381032

Buxbaum, L. J., Schwartz, M. F. & Carew, T. G. (1997). The role of semantic memory in object use. *Cognitive Neuropsychology*, *14*(2), 219-254.

Cabeza, R. & Nyberg, L. (2000). Imaging cognition II: An empirical review of 275 PET and fMRI studies. *J Cogn Neurosci*, *12*(1), 1-47.

Cahn-Weiner, D. A., Boyle, P. A. & Malloy, P. F. (2002). Tests of executive function predict instrumental activities of daily living in community-dwelling older individuals. *Appl Neuropsychol*, *9*(3), 187-191. doi: 10.1207/S15324826AN0903_8

Cahn-Weiner, D. A., Farias, S. T., Julian, L., Harvey, D. J., Kramer, J. H., Reed, B. R., Mungas, D., Wetzel, M. & Chui, H. (2007). Cognitive and neuroimaging predictors of instrumental activities of daily living. *J Int Neuropsychol Soc*, *13*(5), 747-757. doi: 10.1017/S1355617707070853

Cahn-Weiner, D. A., Malloy, P. F., Boyle, P. A., Marran, M. & Salloway, S. (2000). Prediction of functional status from neuropsychological tests in community-dwelling elderly individuals. *Clin Neuropsychol*, *14*(2), 187-195. doi: 10.1076/1385-4046(200005)14:2;1-z;ft187

Cahn-Weiner, D. A., Ready, R. E. & Malloy, P. F. (2003). Neuropsychological predictors of everyday memory and everyday functioning in patients with mild Alzheimer's disease. *J Geriatr Psychiatry Neurol*, *16*(2), 84-89.

Chan, E., MacPherson, S. E., Robinson, G., Turner, M., Lecce, F., Shallice, T. & Cipolotti, L. (2015). Limitations of the trail making test part-B in assessing frontal executive dysfunction. *J Int Neuropsychol Soc*, *21*(2), 169-174. doi: 10.1017/S135561771500003X

Chen, S. T., Sultzer, D. L., Hinkin, C. H., Mahler, M. E. & Cummings, J. L. (1998). Executive dysfunction in Alzheimer's disease: association with neuropsychiatric symptoms and functional impairment. *J Neuropsychiatry Clin Neurosci*, *10*(4), 426-432.

Chow, T. W., Izenberg, A., Binns, M. A., Freedman, M., Stuss, D. T., Scott, C. J., Ramirez, J. & Black, S. E. (2008). Magnetic resonance imaging in frontotemporal dementia shows subcortical atrophy. *Dement Geriatr Cogn Disord*, *26*(1), 79-88. doi: 10.1159/000144028

Corbetta, M., Patel, G. & Shulman, G. L. (2008). The reorienting system of the human brain: from environment to theory of mind. *Neuron*, *58*(3), 306-324. doi: 10.1016/j.neuron.2008.04.017

Cutini, S., Scatturin, P., Menon, E., Bisiacchi, P. S., Gamberini, L., Zorzi, M. & Dell'Acqua, R. (2008). Selective activation of the superior frontal gyrus in task-switching: an event-related fNIRS study. *Neuroimage*, *42*(2), 945-955. doi: 10.1016/j.neuroimage.2008.05.013

du Boisgueheneuc, F., Levy, R., Volle, E., Seassau, M., Duffau, H., Kinkingnehun, S., Samson, Y., S. Zhang & Dubois, B. (2006). Functions of the left superior frontal gyrus in humans: a lesion study. *Brain*, *129*(Pt 12), 3315-3328. doi: 10.1093/brain/awl244

Dubois, B., Slachevsky, A., Litvan, I. & Pillon, B. (2000). The FAB: a Frontal Assessment Battery at bedside. *Neurology*, *55*(11), 1621-1626.
Duncan, J. (1986). Disorganization of behavior after frontal-lobe damage. *Cognitive Neuropsychology*, *3*(3), 271-290. doi: 10.1080/02643298608253360
Farias, S. T., Harrell, E., Neumann, C. & Houtz, A. (2003). The relationship between neuropsychological performance and daily functioning in individuals with Alzheimer's disease: ecological validity of neuropsychological tests. *Archives of Clinical Neuropsychology*, *18*(6), 655-672. doi: http://dx.doi.org/10.1016/S0887-6177(02)00159-2
Frisoni, G. B., Henneman, W. J., Weiner, M. W., Scheltens, P., Vellas, B., Reynish, E., Hudecova J., Hampel H., Burger K., Blennow K., Waldemar G., Johannsen P., Wahlund L. O., Zito G., Rossini P. M., Winblad B., & Barkhof, F. (2008). The pilot European Alzheimer's Disease Neuroimaging Initiative of the European Alzheimer's Disease Consortium. *Alzheimers Dement*, *4*(4), 255-264. doi: 10.1016/ j.jalz.2008.04.009
Fukui, T. & Lee, E. (2009). Visuospatial function is a significant contributor to functional status in patients with Alzheimer's disease. *Am J Alzheimers Dis Other Demen*, *24*(4), 313-321. doi: 10.1177/1533317509333903
Gelinas, I., Gauthier, L., McIntyre, M. & Gauthier, S. (1999). Development of a functional measure for persons with Alzheimer's disease: the disability assessment for dementia. *Am J Occup Ther*, *53*(5), 471-481.
Giovannetti, T., Bettcher, B. M., Brennan, L., Libon, D. J., Burke, M., Duey, K., Nieves, C. & Wambach, D. (2008). Characterization of everyday functioning in mild cognitive impairment: a direct assessment approach. *Dement Geriatr Cogn Disord*, *25*(4), 359-365. doi: 10.1159/000121005
Giovannetti, T., Bettcher, B. M., Brennan, L., Libron, D. J., Kessler, R. K. & Duey, K. (2008). Coffee with jelly or unbuttered toast: commissions and omissions are dissociable aspects of everyday action impairment in Alzheimer's disease. *Neuropsychology*, *22*(2), 235-245. doi: 10.1037/0894-4105.22.2.235
Giovannetti, T., Libon, D. J., Buxbaum, L. J. & Schwartz, M. F. (2002). Naturalistic action impairments in dementia. *Neuropsychologia*, *40*(8), 1220-1232.
Giovannetti, T., Schmidt, K. S., Gallo, J. L., Sestito, N. & Libon, D. J. (2006). Everyday action in dementia: evidence for differential deficits in Alzheimer's disease versus subcortical vascular dementia. *J Int Neuropsychol Soc*, *12*(1), 45-53. doi: 10.1017/s1355617706060012

Giovannetti, T., Schwartz, M. F. & Buxbaum, L. J. (2007). The Coffee Challenge: a new method for the study of everyday action errors. *J Clin Exp Neuropsychol, 29*(7), 690-705. doi: 10.1080/13803390600932286

Glosser, G., Gallo, J., Duda, N., de Vries, J. J., Clark, C. M. & Grossman, M. (2002). Visual perceptual functions predict instrumental activities of daily living in patients with dementia. *Neuropsychiatry Neuropsychol Behav Neurol, 15*(3), 198-206.

Grigsby, J., Kaye, K., Baxter, J., Shetterly, S. M. & Hamman, R. F. (1998). Executive cognitive abilities and functional status among community-dwelling older persons in the San Luis Valley Health and Aging Study. *J Am Geriatr Soc, 46*(5), 590-596.

Hartmann, K., Goldenberg, G., Daumüller, M. & Hermsdörfer, J. (2005). It takes the whole brain to make a cup of coffee: the neuropsychology of naturalistic actions involving technical devices. *Neuropsychologia, 43*(4), 625-637. doi: http://dx.doi.org/10.1016/j.neuropsychologia.2004.07.015

Herholz, K., Schopphoff, H., Schmidt, M., Mielke, R., Eschner, W., Scheidhauer, K., . . . Ebmeier, K. (2002). Direct comparison of spatially normalized PET and SPECT scans in Alzheimer's disease. *J Nucl Med, 43*(1), 21-26.

Hill, R. D., Backman, L. & Fratiglioni, L. (1995). Determinants of functional abilities in dementia. *J Am Geriatr Soc, 43*(10), 1092-1097.

Hodges, J. R. & Patterson, K. (1995). Is semantic memory consistently impaired early in the course of Alzheimer's disease? Neuroanatomical and diagnostic implications. *Neuropsychologia, 33*(4), 441-459.

Jefferson, A. L., Barakat, L. P., Giovannetti, T., Paul, R. H. & Glosser, G. (2006). Object perception impairments predict instrumental activities of daily living dependence in Alzheimer's disease. *J Clin Exp Neuropsychol, 28*(6), 884-897. doi: 10.1080/13803390591001034

Lanctot, K. L., Moosa, S., Herrmann, N., Leibovitch, F. S., Rothenburg, L., Cotter, A. & Black, S. E. (2007). A SPECT study of apathy in Alzheimer's disease. *Dement Geriatr Cogn Disord, 24*(1), 65-72. doi: 10.1159/000103633

Landau, S. M., Harvey, D., Madison, C. M., Koeppe, R. A., Reiman, E. M., Foster, N. L., Weiner M. W., Jagust W. J.;. Alzheimer's Disease Neuroimaging, I. (2011). Associations between cognitive, functional, and FDG-PET measures of decline in AD and MCI. *Neurobiol Aging, 32*(7), 1207-1218. doi: 10.1016/j.neurobiolaging.2009.07.002

Lawton, M. P. & Brody, E. M. (1969). Assessment of older people: self-maintaining and instrumental activities of daily living. *Gerontologist, 9*(3), 179-186.

Lewis, M. S. & Miller, L. S. (2007). Executive control functioning and functional ability in older adults. *Clin Neuropsychol, 21*(2), 274-285. doi: 10.1080/13854040500519752

Libon, D., Schmidt, K. S., Gallo, J. L., Penney, D. L., Swenson, R., Giovannetti, T. & Miller, J. A. (2005). The prototypicality of extra-list intrusion errors produced on a serial list-learning task by patients with mild dementia. [Abstract] *Journal of the International Neuropsychological Society, 11*(Suppl. 1), 92-93.

Loewenstein, D. A., Rubert, M. P., Arguelles, T. & Duara, R. (1995). Neuropsychological test performance and prediction of functional capacities among Spanish-speaking and English-speaking patients with dementia. *Arch Clin Neuropsychol, 10*(2), 75-88.

Mahurin, R. K., DeBettignies, B. H. & Pirozzolo, F. J. (1991). Structured assessment of independent living skills: preliminary report of a performance measure of functional abilities in dementia. *J Gerontol, 46*(2), P58-66.

Majdandzic, J., Grol, M. J., van Schie, H. T., Verhagen, L., Toni, I. & Bekkering, H. (2007). The role of immediate and final goals in action planning: an fMRI study. *Neuroimage, 37*(2), 589-598. doi: 10.1016/j.neuroimage.2007.04.071

Manandhar, M. C. (1995). Functional ability and nutritional status of free-living elderly people. *Proc Nutr Soc, 54*(3), 677-691.

Marshall, G. A., Monserratt, L., Harwood, D., Mandelkern, M., Cummings, J. L. & Sultzer, D. L. (2007). Positron emission tomography metabolic correlates of apathy in Alzheimer disease. *Arch Neurol, 64*(7), 1015-1020. doi: 10.1001/archneur.64.7.1015

Marshall, G. A., Rentz, D. M., Frey, M. T., Locascio, J. J., Johnson, K. A., Sperling, R. A. & Alzheimer's Disease Neuroimaging, I. (2011). Executive function and instrumental activities of daily living in mild cognitive impairment and Alzheimer's disease. *Alzheimers Dement, 7*(3), 300-308. doi: 10.1016/j.jalz.2010.04.005

Martino, J., Gabarros, A., Deus, J., Juncadella, M., Acebes, J. J., Torres, A. & Pujol, J. (2011). Intrasurgical mapping of complex motor function in the superior frontal gyrus. *Neuroscience, 179*, 131-142. doi: 10.1016/j.neuroscience.2011.01.047

Martyr, A. & Clare, L. (2012). Executive function and activities of daily living in Alzheimer's disease: a correlational meta-analysis. *Dement Geriatr Cogn Disord*, *33*(2-3), 189-203. doi: 10.1159/000338233

McDonald, C. R., McEvoy, L. K., Gharapetian, L., Fennema-Notestine, C., Hagler, D. J., Jr., Holland, D., Koyama A., Brewer J. B. Dale, A. M. (2009). Regional rates of neocortical atrophy from normal aging to early Alzheimer disease. *Neurology*, *73*(6), 457-465. doi: 10.1212/ WNL.0b013e3181b16431

Melrose, R. J., Ettenhofer, M. L., Harwood, D., Achamallah, N., Campa, O., Mandelkern, M. & Sultzer, D. L. (2011). Cerebral metabolism, cognition, and functional abilities in Alzheimer disease. *J Geriatr Psychiatry Neurol*, *24*(3), 127-134. doi: 10.1177/0891988711405333

Mesulam, M. (2000). Behavioral Neuroanatomy. Large-Scale Networks, Association Cortex, Frontal Syndromes, the Limbic System, and Hemispheric Specializations. In M. Mesulam (Ed.), *Principles of Behavioural and Congitive Neurology* (2nd ed.). New York: Oxford University Press

Migneco, O., Benoit, M., Koulibaly, P. M., Dygai, I., Bertogliati, C., Desvignes, P., Robert, P. H., Malandain G., Bussiere F. & Darcourt, J. (2001). Perfusion brain SPECT and statistical parametric mapping analysis indicate that apathy is a cingulate syndrome: a study in Alzheimer's disease and nondemented patients. *Neuroimage*, *13*(5), 896-902. doi: 10.1006/nimg.2000.0741

Millan-Calenti, J. C., Tubio, J., Pita-Fernandez, S., Rochette, S., Lorenzo, T. & Maseda, A. (2012). Cognitive impairment as predictor of functional dependence in an elderly sample. *Arch Gerontol Geriatr*, *54*(1), 197-201. doi: 10.1016/j.archger.2011.02.010

Minoshima, S., Giordani, B., Berent, S., Frey, K. A., Foster, N. L. & Kuhl, D. E. (1997). Metabolic reduction in the posterior cingulate cortex in very early Alzheimer's disease. *Ann Neurol*, *42*(1), 85-94.

Mioshi, E., Dawson, K., Mitchell, J., Arnold, R. & Hodges, J. R. (2006). The Addenbrooke's Cognitive Examination Revised (ACE-R): a brief cognitive test battery for dementia screening. *Int J Geriatr Psychiatry*, *21*(11), 1078-1085. doi: 10.1002/gps.1610

Mioshi, E., Hodges, J. R. & Hornberger, M. (2013). Neural correlates of activities of daily living in frontotemporal dementia. *J Geriatr Psychiatry Neurol*, *26*(1), 51-57. doi: 10.1177/0891988713477474

Mioshi, E., Kipps, C. M., Dawson, K., Mitchell, J., Graham, A. & Hodges, J. R. (2007). Activities of daily living in frontotemporal dementia and

Alzheimer disease. *Neurology*, *68*(24), 2077-2084. doi: 10.1212/ 01.wnl.0000264897.13722.53

Myers, A. M., Holliday, P. J., Harvey, K. A. & Hutchinson, K. S. (1993). Functional performance measures: are they superior to self-assessments? *J Gerontol*, *48*(5), M196-206.

Nadkarni, N. K., Levy-Cooperman, N. & Black, S. E. (2012). Functional correlates of instrumental activities of daily living in mild Alzheimer's disease. *Neurobiol Aging*, *33*(1), 53-60. doi: 10.1016/ j.neurobiolaging. 2010.02.001

Nobili, F., Copello, F., Buffoni, F., Vitali, P., Girtler, N., Bordoni, C., . . . Rodriguez, G. (2001). Regional cerebral blood flow and prognostic evaluation in Alzheimer's disease. *Dement Geriatr Cogn Disord*, *12*(2), 89-97. doi: 51241

Ochipa, C., Rothi, L. J. & Heilman, K. M. (1989). Ideational apraxia: a deficit in tool selection and use. *Ann Neurol*, *25*(2), 190-193. doi: 10.1002/ana.410250214

Ott, B. R., Heindel, W. C., Whelihan, W. M., Caron, M. D., Piatt, A. L. & Noto, R. B. (2000). A single-photon emission computed tomography imaging study of driving impairment in patients with Alzheimer's disease. *Dement Geriatr Cogn Disord*, *11*(3), 153-160. doi: 17229

Ott, B. R., Lafleche, G., Whelihan, W. M., Buongiorno, G. W., Albert, M. S. & Fogel, B. S. (1996). Impaired awareness of deficits in Alzheimer disease. *Alzheimer Dis Assoc Disord*, *10*(2), 68-76.

Pa, J., Possin, K. L., Wilson, S. M., Quitania, L. C., Kramer, J. H., Boxer, A. L., Weiner, M.W. & Johnson, J. K. (2010). Gray matter correlates of set-shifting among neurodegenerative disease, mild cognitive impairment, and healthy older adults. *J Int Neuropsychol Soc*, *16*(4), 640-650. doi: 10.1017/ S1355617710000408

Phillips, A. G. & Carr, G. D. (1987). Cognition and the basal ganglia: a possible substrate for procedural knowledge. *Can J Neurol Sci*, *14*(3 Suppl), 381-385.

Ragozzino, M. E. (2007). The contribution of the medial prefrontal cortex, orbitofrontal cortex, and dorsomedial striatum to behavioral flexibility. *Ann N Y Acad Sci*, *1121*, 355-375.

Rowe, J. B. & Passingham, R. E. (2001). Working memory for location and time: activity in prefrontal area 46 relates to selection rather than maintenance in memory. *Neuroimage*, *14*(1 Pt 1), 77-86.

Rusted, J. & Sheppard, L. (2002). Action-based memory in Alzheimer's disease: a longitudinal look at tea making. *Neurocase*, *8*(1-2), 111-126. doi: 10.1093/neucas/8.1.111

Salmon, E., Lespagnard, S., Marique, P., Peeters, F., Herholz, K., Perani, D., Holthoff V., Kalbe E., Anchisi D., Adam S., Collette F. & Garraux, G. (2005). Cerebral metabolic correlates of four dementia scales in Alzheimer's disease. *J Neurol*, *252*(3), 283-290. doi: 10.1007/s00415-005-0551-3

Schmitter-Edgecombe, M., Parsey, C. & Cook, D. J. (2011). Cognitive correlates of functional performance in older adults: comparison of self-report, direct observation, and performance-based measures. *J Int Neuropsychol Soc*, *17*(5), 853-864. doi: 10.1017/s1355617711000865

Schmitter-Edgecombe, M. & Parsey, C. M. (2014). Assessment of Functional Change and Cognitive Correlates in the Progression From Healthy Cognitive Aging to Dementia. *Neuropsychology*, *28*(6), 881-893. doi: 10.1037/neu0000109

Schwartz, M. F., Buxbaum, L. J., Ferraro, M., Veramonti, T. & Segal, M. (2002). *NAT: Naturalistic Action Test: Manual.* Bury St. Edmunds, UK: Thames Valley Test Company.

Schwartz, M. F., Buxbaum, L. J., Montgomery, M. W., Fitzpatrick-DeSalme, E., Hart, T., Ferraro, M., Lee, S. S & Coslett, H. B. (1999). Naturalistic action production following right hemisphere stroke. *Neuropsychologia*, *37*(1), 51-66.

Schwartz, M. F., Montgomery, M. W., Buxbaum, L. J., Lee, S. S., Carew, T. G., Coslett, H. B., Ferraro M., Fitzpatrick-DeSalme E., Hart T. & Mayer, N. (1998). Naturalistic action impairment in closed head injury. *Neuropsychology*, *12*(1), 13-28.

Smith, E. E. & Jonides, J. (1999). Storage and executive processes in the frontal lobes. *Science*, *283*(5408), 1657-1661.

Sultzer, D. L., Mahler, M. E., Mandelkern, M. A., Cummings, J. L., Van Gorp, W. G., Hinkin, C. H. & Berisford, M. A. (1995). The relationship between psychiatric symptoms and regional cortical metabolism in Alzheimer's disease. *J Neuropsychiatry Clin Neurosci*, *7*(4), 476-484.

Tam, C. W., Lam, L. C., Chiu, H. F. & Lui, V. W. (2007). Characteristic profiles of instrumental activities of daily living in Chinese older persons with mild cognitive impairment. *Am J Alzheimers Dis Other Demen*, *22*(3), 211-217. doi: 10.1177/1533317507301597

Tulving, E. (1983). *Elements of Episodic Memory.* New York: Oxford University Press.

Vidoni, E. D., Honea, R. A. & Burns, J. M. (2010). Neural correlates of impaired functional independence in early Alzheimer's disease. *J Alzheimers Dis*, *19*(2), 517-527. doi: 10.3233/JAD-2010-1245

Vogel, A., Gade, A., Stokholm, J. & Waldemar, G. (2005). Semantic memory impairment in the earliest phases of Alzheimer's disease. *Dement Geriatr Cogn Disord*, *19*(2-3), 75-81. doi: DEM20050192_3075 [pii] 10.1159/000082352

Wechsler, D. (1945). A standardized memory scale for clinical use. . *Journal of Psychology*, *19*, 97-95.

Wechsler, D. (1981). *Manual for the Wechsler Adult Intelligence Scale—Revised (WAIS-R).* San Antonio, TX: The Psychological Corporation.

Willis, S. & Marsiske, M. (1993). *Manual for the Everyday Problems Test.* University Park, PA: Department of Human Development and Family Studies, Pennsylvania State University.

In: Activities of Daily Living (ADL)
Editor: Scott T. Lively

ISBN: 978-1-63463-913-2

Chapter 2

Activities of Daily Living, Activities Parallel to Daily Living, and Disease-Specific Quality of Life in Patients with Knee Osteoarthritis

Kazuki Hirao,* PhD, OTR
Department of Occupational Therapy,
School of Health Science and Social Welfare,
Kibi International University, Takahashi, Okayama, Japan

Abstract

The incidence of age-related degenerative musculoskeletal disease is increasing in much of the industrialized world due to population aging. Knee osteoarthritis (OA) is one of the most common diseases in this category. Although not a disease that directly affects short-term survival, knee OA nonetheless negatively impacts essential activities of daily living (ADLs), activities parallel to daily living(APDLs), and general

* Address: 8 Iga-machi Takahashi, Okayama 716-8508, Japan; Email Address: hirao-k@kiui.ac.jp.

quality of life (QOL).Moreover, knee OA patients with limited mobility (sedentary) may be at greater risk of early mortality due to metabolic and cardiovascular diseases. First, this chapterdiscussesthe prevalence of knee OA, the various diagnostic tools used, and the physical and psychological sequelaethat influence disease-specific QOL. Second, the correlations amongADLs, APDLs, and disease-specific QOL are discussed. Finally, survey results onfrequenciesof disease-specific difficulties in ADLs (e.g., dressing the lower body, going to the toilet, and climbing stairs) and APDLs (e.g., cooking, washing, and cleaning) are presented. A significant fraction of knee OA patients who have maintained functional independence still experience difficulty with these daily tasks.

Introduction

Osteoarthritis (OA) is a disease characterized by progressive cartilage degeneration, resulting in localized pain and limited functional motility. Knee OA is the most frequent subtype [1] and is particularly prevalent in the elderly.Incidence of knee OA increases rapidly after the age of 50and more than 80% of the population 60 years and older exhibit some signs of knee OA on X-ray [2]. Approximately40% of those older than 60 years show some knee OA symptoms,and knee OA is an obstacle to their daily life in approximately 10% of this age group [2]. Thus, knee OA is a common malady of aging and is likely to reduce healthy life expectancy. In addition, it is associated with both lost productivity in the labor force and rising healthcare costs.

Locomotive syndrome refers to a state of immobility currently requiring nursing care or that confers an increased probability of needing such care in the futuredue to progressive failure of the musculoskeletal system [3]. A major goal of preventive care measures promotion in Japan is a greater understanding ofthe pathology, prevention, and treatment of locomotive syndrome [3], of which knee OA is among the most common causes [3].

Risk factors of knee OA includeolder age, female gender, past history of knee injury,and obesity [4]. In one study, 123 out of 140 total knee arthroplasty patients had a previous meniscal injury [5]. In addition, reduced bone mineral density [6], knee extensor muscleweakness [7, 8], and mild cognitive impairment are common in knee OA [9]. In fact, the presence of knee OA is associated with a 4.9-fold increase in the incidence of mild cognitive impairment compared to age-matched controls [9]. Studies have also found a significant association between knee OA and metabolic syndrome [10, 11].

Assessment of Knee Osteoarthritis

1. Kellgren-Lawrence Grading

Typically, knee OA is diagnosed by X-ray. The Kellgren-Lawrence classification has been used for decades to grade knee OA severity [12]. As cartilage disappears, the joint space narrows and residual cartilage thickness can be estimated from the joint bone gap on X-ray. On X-rays acquired in a lying position, however, the joint space is often enlarged even in the presence of cartilage damage. Therefore, to accurately estimate the extent of cartilage damage, X-rays are acquired while applying weight in the standing position. The Kellgren-Lawrence grading system classifies knee OA from anterioposterior X-rays on a scale from 0 to IV: 0 (no evidence of OA), I (doubtful), II(minimal), III(moderate), or IV (severe) [12]. Specifically, grade 0 indicates normal joint structure, grade Iindicates slight osteophyte formation or subchondral bone hardening but no joint space narrowing,grade II indicates joint space narrowing ≤25% and obvious osteophyte formation,grade III indicates joint narrowing of 50%–75% and formation of multiple osteophytes, and grade IV indicates joint space narrowing ≥75% with bone deformity and large osteophytes [12].

2. Magnetic Resonance Imaging (MRI)

Using 1.5T (or stronger) MRI, it is possible to assess changes in intra-articular structures in greater detail than is possible by conventional X-ray[13].Knee OA severity is graded semiquantitatively by MRI according to the Whole-Organ Magnetic Resonance Imaging Score (WORMS) [14].The WORMS includes additional evaluation items, such as cartilage abrasion, half-moon damage, and bone marrow abnormality. While semiquantitative, the WORMS shows high inter-rater agreement [14].

3. Strength Evaluation of Knee Joint Muscles

The strength of muscles associated with knee movement is commonly evaluated using manual muscle testing (MMT), where a grade of 5is "Normal" muscle strength, 4is "Good," 3is "Fair," 2 is "Poor," 1is "Trace,"and 0 indicates no appreciable strength [15]. Infrequent joint movement can cause muscle atrophy, as one study reported a significant 22% decrease in quadriceps strength of patients with radiologic OA compared to the control group [16]. In contrast, another study reported that quadriceps muscle strength in early knee OA did not differ significantly from controls [17].

4. Five-Meter Walk Test (5MWT)

The 5MWT is widely used as an indicator of walking ability [18] as it is a simple test that does not require a large space or special equipment. All that is required is a straight indoor 11-m walking path with marks at the 3-m and 8-m points to measure the 5-m walking speed using a stopwatch.

5. Functional Reach Test (FRT)

The FRT has been used as an indicator of dynamic balance ability [19] and the reliability and validity of this test have been established [19, 20]. The FRT evaluates balance by having the standing patient stretch out a hand as far as possible with the arm at 90° flexion without stepping forward. The primary measure is the difference (in cm) between the initial and final hand position in the horizontal plane.

6. Functional Independence Measure (FIM)

The FIM is a common grading system for evaluation of basic activities of daily living (ADLs). The self-report questionnaire consists of 18 items (13 motor items and 5 cognitive items) for evaluation of actual daily activities. Overall function is then graded in 7 levels. Subscores range from 13−91 points for motor function and 5−35 points for cognitive function, with the highest possible total score being 126 points (total functional independence) and the lowest score being 18 points (severe limitation on functional independence) [21].

7. Western Ontario and McMaster Universities Osteoarthritis Index (WOMAC)

The WOMAC is a disease-specific, self-reported health-related quality of life (QOL) index assessed using either a 5-point Likert scale or Visual Analog Scale (VAS) [22, 23], with 100 points indicating the best possible QOL and 0 points the worst. The WOMAC measures five items for pain, two for stiffness, and 17 for functional limitation.

8. Japanese Knee Osteoarthritis Measure (JKOM)

The JKOM consists of 25 questions covering the following four subscales: "Pain and stiffness of the knees" (8 items), "Condition in daily life" (10 items), "General activities" (5 items), and "Health condition" (2 items) [24]. Each item is multiplechoice and the patient selects an answer ranging from the best (1 point) to the worst condition (5 points) [24]. Self-evaluation of the severity of knee pain is done using a VAS. The reliability and validity of the JKOM have been verifiedand factor analysis distinguished three domains: pain, mobility limitation for activities of daily life, and limitation of social and health-related activities [24].

Conservative Treatment of Knee OA

The most common conservative treatments for knee OA are patient education, weight loss, and therapeutic exercise.

Therapeutic Exercise

A previous meta-analysis suggested that land-based therapeutic exercise for knee OA patients is effective for reducing knee pain and improving physical function [25].Quadriceps and lower limb muscle strengthening exercises alleviated the pain at rest and after surgery and improved range of motion, muscle strength, and QOL [26].Another study reported thataerobic exercise (walking, underwater running, yoga, Tai chi chuan) significantly alleviated resting pain and joint pain on pressure and improved both knee function and range of motion [27].

Education for Patients and Educational Guidance

A patient education program using lectures and discussions led to reduced pain, improved quadriceps muscle strength, and higher WOMAC scores [28]. Moreover, enforcement of the self-administration program facilitated improvement and reduced medical expenses [29].

Weight Reduction

Combined diet and exercise intervention in older adults with knee OA had a positive effect on health-related QOL compared to an age-matched control knee OA group [30].Exercise and dietary weight loss interventions improved the stair climb, 6-minute walk performance, and mobility-related self-efficacy in overweight and obese older adults with knee OA [31].

Body Function, Mind Function, and Disease-Specific QOL

Here, I summarize results of our own studies [32, 33].

Study participants were 38 women diagnosed with bilateral knee OA by clinical and X-ray findings. Patients with cerebrovascular disease, leg fracture, or a history of surgery were excluded, and only those who scored 21 points or more on the Hasegawa Dementia Scale-Revised (HDS-R) were enrolled as a score ≤ 20is indicative of dementia independent of educational level [34]. Mean age was 77.3 ± 7.1 years, height was 147.1 ± 8 cm, body weight was 51.3 ± 9.5 kg, and body mass index (BMI) was 23.6 ± 3.6 kg/m^2. With respect to the classification of knee OA duration, 15 patients were grade II, 16 patients were grade III, and 7 patients were grade IV, so 80% of the patients were in either grade II or III.

Positive correlations were observed between the BMI and JKOM scores, suggesting that excess weight/obesity is an aggravating factor in knee OA that has a negative impact on QOL. Therefore, diet and exercise programs are essential for these patients.

Correlations were also observed between the JKOM score and both the FRT and 5MWT, indicating that the degree of physical function affects QOL. As FRT and 5MWT are easily measured, they are possible convenient indices for predicting QOL in knee OA patients. In addition, correlations were observed between the pain-related VAS and the JKOM scores [24]. Therefore, not surprisingly, knee pain adversely affects QOL of knee OA patients.

In contrast, there was no significant correlation between the Geriatric Depression Scale (GDS) score, widely used in the evaluation of depression in the elderly [35], and the JKOM in the entire patient cohort. However, a correlation was observed between GDS and JKOM scores in the depressed subgroup (n = 19). Further analysis revealed that this correlation was due to a strong correlation between the JKOM subscale "Condition in daily life" and the GDS.

Correlations were not observed between the severity on X-ray and JKOM score. Moreover, correlations were also not observed between the severity on X-ray and clinical outcome [36, 37].Therefore, severity on the X-ray does not necessarily associate with negative impact on QOL. Rather, individual differences in functional outcome (pain, functional impairment) were strongly dependent on psychological factors [36].

ADLs, APDLs, and Disease-Specific QOL

I used FIM [21] as an index of ADLs in this study [33]. FIM Motor Items were investigated in this study and participants who scored 6 or 7 points were defined as the independent subgroup. To investigate the proportion of the independent subgroup reporting difficulties in ADLs, questions from the JKOM "Condition in daily life" were employed: [(Q-9) How difficult is ascending or descending stairs? (Q-11) How difficult is standing up from sitting on a Western-style toilet? (Q-12) How difficult is to wear pants, skirts, and underwear? (Q-13) Howdifficult is putting on socks?]. These questions correspond to some of the FIM motor items (i.e., Dressing-lower body, Transferring to toilet, and Ascending/Descending stairs). The answers to questions 9−13 were selected from among the following options: (1) Not at all difficult; (2) A little difficult; (3) Moderately difficult; (4) Quite difficult; and

(5) Extremely difficult. Patients answering (2) to (5) were considered to have difficulty with that particular task.

The mean ± standard deviation JKOM score of the entire cohort was 64.9 ± 19.7 points and JKOM subscores were 21.2 ± 7.3 for "Pain and stiffness of the knees," 24.6 ± 8.6 for "Condition in daily life," 14.4 ± 4.8 for "General activities," and 4.6 ± 1.9 for "Health condition."

Negative correlations were observed between the FIM motor items score and the JKOM total score and between the FIM motor items score and all JKOM subscores. Thus, a lower JKOM total score was indicative of higher QOL, indicating that patients with more independence in ADLs enjoyed a higher QOL. Therefore, improvement of ADLs has a positive influence on QOL.

We also analyzed the frequency of subjective difficulties in performing three specific critical ADLs–Dressing-lower body, Transferring to the toilet, and Ascending/descending stairs–among the independent participants. Almost all of the participants were independent (97.3%, n = 37); however, 48.6% (n = 18) of the independent patients still reported difficulty in putting on/taking off trousers, skirts, and pants, while 56.8% (n = 21) reported difficulty putting on or removing socks. A restricted range of knee motion may cause difficulty when reaching down to grasp a pair of trousers, or a patient may feel unsteady due to muscle weakness and/or pain. All 38 (100%) of the participants were independent for toilet transfer, but 47.4% (n = 18) still reported difficulty rising from a Western-style toilet. Similarly, a previous study reported that 44% (n = 114) of patients with knee OA had difficulty or were unable to get up from a chair[38], which is compatible with our results. In contrast, only 63.2% (n = 24) of the participants were independent for stair-climbing and91.7% (n = 22) of the independent patients reported difficulty ascending and/or descending stairs. Ascending and descending stairs imposes a greater load on the knees than walking on a flat surface. In fact, the load rises to approximately four times body weight, thereby explaining why most otherwise independent patients reported difficulty with stairs [39].A previously study reported difficulty climbing and descend stairs in 62% and 83% of 114 patients with knee OA, respectively [38]. The higher percentage of patients reporting difficulty in our study is probably due to inclusion of patients with bilateral knee OA.

To go to a beauty salon:29% (n = 11) of the participants felt that it was difficult to go to a beauty salon.

Cooking a simple meal: 34.3% (n = 13) of the participants felt that it was difficult to cook a simple meal.

Cooking an elaborate meal: 36.8% (n = 14) of the participants felt that it was difficult to cook an elaborate meal.

Washing clothes: 15.8% (n = 6) of the participants felt that it was difficult to wash clothes.

Drying clothes: 39.5% (n = 15) of the participants felt that it was difficult to dry clothes.

Cleaning up after cooking: 23.7% (n = 9) of the participants felt that it was difficult cleaning after cooking.

Cleaning the bathtub: 60.5% (n = 23) of the participants felt that it was difficult to clean the bathtub.

Cleaning the washroom: 44.7% (n = 17) of the participants felt that it was difficult to clean the washroom.

Collecting the garbage: 28.9% (n = 11) of the participants felt that it was difficult to collect the garbage.

Taking out the garbage: 47.4% (n = 18) of the participants felt that it was difficult to take out the garbage.

Thus, a substantial minority of patients expressed difficulties in specific APDLs, "higher order" activities that nonetheless contribute to QOL. Unexpectedly, percentages were lower than for the three major ADLs, possibly because these APDLs are group activities involving families while essential ADLs are private activities.

It can be assumed that difficulty in ADLs places a heavy physical and mental burden on independent knee OA patients. In the clinical setting, both objective ADLs and subjective (patient-oriented) QOL should be evaluated. It is important to decide on the appropriate intervention based on the results of such evaluations.

References

[1] Muraki S, Oka H, Akune T, Mabuchi A, En-yo Y, Yoshida M, Saika A, Suzuki T, Yoshida H, Ishibashi H, Yamamoto S, Nakamura K, Kawaguchi H, Yoshimura N. Prevalence of radiographic knee osteoarthritis and its association with knee painin the elderly of Japanese population-based cohorts: the ROAD study. *Osteoarthr. Cartilage* 2009; 17(9): 1137-43.

[2] Chamberlain MA, Care G, Harfield B. Physiotherapy in osteoarthrosis of the knees. A controlled trial of hospital versus home exercises. *Int. Rehabil. Med.*1982;4(2):101-6.

[3] Nakamura K. The concept and treatment of locomotive syndrome: its acceptance and spread in Japan. *J. Orthop. Sci.* 2011;16(5):489-91.

[4] Blagojevic M, Jinks C, Jeffery A, Jordan KP. Risk factors for onset ofosteoarthritis of the knee in older adults: a systematic review andmeta-analysis. *Osteoarthr. Cartilage* 2010;18(1):24-33.

[5] Chan WP, Huang GS, Hsu SM, Chang YC, Ho WP. Radiographic joint space narrowing in osteoarthritis of the knee: relationship to meniscal tears and duration of pain. *Skeletal Radiol.* 2008;37(10):917-22.

[6] Sudo A, Miyamoto N, Horikawa K, Urawa M, Yamakawa T, Yamada T, Uchida A. Prevalence and risk factors for knee osteoarthritis in elderly Japanese men and women. *J. Orthop. Sci.* 2008;13(5):413-8.

[7] Yoshimura N, Muraki S, Oka H, Kawaguchi H, Nakamura K, Akune T. Cohortprofile: research on Osteoarthritis/Osteoporosis Against Disability study. *Int. J. Epidemiol.* 2010;39(4):988-95.

[8] Yoshimura N, Muraki S, Oka H, Mabuchi A, En-Yo Y, Yoshida M, Saika A, Yoshida H, Suzuki T, Yamamoto S, Ishibashi H, Kawaguchi H, Nakamura K, Akune T.Prevalence of knee osteoarthritis, lumbar spondylosis, and osteoporosis in Japanese men and women: the research on osteoarthritis/osteoporosis against disability study. *J. Bone Miner. Metab.* 2009;27(5):620-8.

[9] Yoshimura N, Muraki S, Oka H, Kawaguchi H, Nakamura K, Tanaka S, Akune T. Does mild cognitive impairment affect the occurrence of radiographic knee osteoarthritis? A 3-year follow-up in the ROAD study. *BMJ Open.* 2012;2(6):e001520.

[10] Yoshimura N, Muraki S, Oka H, Kawaguchi H, Nakamura K, Akune T. Association of knee osteoarthritis with the accumulation of metabolic risk factors such as overweight, hypertension, dyslipidemia, and impaired glucose tolerance in Japanese men and women: the ROAD study. *J. Rheumatol.* 2011;38(5):921-30.

[11] Yoshimura N, Muraki S, Oka H, Tanaka S, Kawaguchi H, Nakamura K, Akune T. Accumulation of metabolic risk factors such as overweight, hypertension, dyslipidaemia, and impaired glucose tolerance raises the risk of occurrence and progression of knee osteoarthritis: a 3-year follow-up of the ROAD study. *Osteoarthr. Cartilage* 2012;20(11):1217-26.

[12] Kellgren JH, Lawrence JS. Radiological assessment of osteo-arthrosis. *Ann. Rheum. Dis.* 1957;16(4):494-502.

[13] 13. Javaid MK, Lynch JA, Tolstykh I, Guermazi A, Roemer F, Aliabadi P, McCullochC, Curtis J, Felson D, Lane NE, Torner J, Nevitt M. Pre-radiographic MRI findings are associated with onset of knee symptoms: the most study. *Osteoarthr. Cartilage* 2010;18(3):323-8.

[14] Peterfy CG, Guermazi A, Zaim S, Tirman PF, Miaux Y, White D, Kothari M, Lu Y, Fye K, Zhao S, Genant HK. Whole-Organ Magnetic Resonance Imaging Score (WORMS) of the knee in osteoarthritis. *Osteoarthr. Cartilage* 2004;12(3):177-90.

[15] Hislop H, Avers D, Brown M.Daniels and Worthingham's Muscle Testing: Techniques of Manual Examination and Performance Testing. New York, USA: *Elsevier* Ink.; 2013.

[16] Palmieri-Smith RM, Thomas AC, Karvonen-Gutierrez C, Sowers MF. Isometric quadriceps strength in women with mild, moderate, and severe knee osteoarthritis. *Am. J. Phys. Med. Rehabil.* 2010;89(7):541-8.

[17] Thomas AC, Sowers M, Karvonen-Gutierrez C, Palmieri-Smith RM. Lack of quadriceps dysfunction in women with early knee osteoarthritis. *J. Orthop. Res.*2010;28(5):595-9.

[18] Salbach NM, Mayo NE, Higgins J, Ahmed S, Finch LE, Richards CL. Responsiveness and predictability of gait speed and other disability measures in acute stroke. *Arch. Phys. Med. Rehabil.* 2001;82(9):1204-12.

[19] Duncan PW, Weiner DK, Chandler J, Studenski S. Functional reach: a new clinical measure of balance. *J. Gerontol.* 1990;45(6):M192-7.

[20] 20. Duncan PW, Studenski S, Chandler J, Prescott B. Functional reach: predictive validity in a sample of elderly male veterans. *J. Gerontol.* 1992;47(3):M93-8.

[21] Keith RA, Granger CV, Hamilton BB, Sherwin FS. The functional independence measure: a new tool for rehabilitation. *Adv. Clin. Rehabil.* 1987;1:6-18.

[22] Bellamy N, Buchanan WW, Goldsmith CH, Campbell J, Stitt LW. Validation study of WOMAC: a health status instrument for measuring clinically important patient relevant outcomes to antirheumatic drug therapy in patients with osteoarthritis of the hip or knee. *J. Rheumatol.* 1988;15(12):1833-40.

[23] Bellamy N, Buchanan WW, Goldsmith CH, Campbell J: Validation study of WOMAC: a health status instrument for measuring clinically

important patient relevant outcomes following total hip or knee arthroplasty in osteoarthritis. *J. Orthop. Rheumatol.* 1988;1:95-108.

[24] Akai M, Doi T, Fujino K, Iwaya T, Kurosawa H, Nasu T. An outcome measure for Japanese people with knee osteoarthritis. *J. Rheumatol.* 2005;32(8):1524-32.

[25] Fransen M, McConnell S, Harmer AR, Van der Esch M, Simic M, Bennell KL. Exercise for osteoarthritis of the knee. *Cochrane Database Syst. Rev*. 2015;1:CD004376.

[26] Lange AK, Vanwanseele B, Fiatarone Singh MA. Strength training for treatment of osteoarthritis of the knee: a systematic review. *Arthritis Rheum.* 2008;59(10):1488-94.

[27] Brosseau L, Pelland L, Wells G, Macleay L, Lamothe C, Michaud G, Lambert J, Robinson V, Tugwell P. Efficacy of aerobic exercises for osteoarthritis (part II): a meta-analysis. *Phys Ther. Rev*. 2004;9(3):125-145.

[28] Maurer BT, Stern AG, Kinossian B, Cook KD, Schumacher HR Jr. Osteoarthritis of the knee: isokinetic quadriceps exercise versus an educational intervention. Arch Phys Med Rehabil. 1999;80(10):1293-9.

[29] Jessep SA, Walsh NE, Ratcliffe J, Hurley MV. Long-term clinical benefits and costs of an integrated rehabilitation programme compared without patient physiotherapy for chronic knee pain. *Physiotherapy* 2009;95(2):94-102.

[30] Rejeski WJ, Focht BC, Messier SP, Morgan T, Pahor M, Penninx B. Obese, older adults with knee osteoarthritis: weight loss, exercise, and quality of life. *Health Psychol.* 2002;21(5):419-26.

[31] Focht BC, Rejeski WJ, Ambrosius WT, Katula JA, Messier SP. Exercise, self-efficacy, and mobility performance in overweight and obese older adults with knee osteoarthritis. *Arthritis Rheum.* 2005;53(5):659-65.

[32] Hirao K, Okishima K, Numata K, Tomokuni Y, Ogura T, Shimada K: Analysis of the effect of physical limitations and depression on quality of life (QOL) in patients with symptomatic osteoarthritis of the knees: Use of the Japanese Knee Osteoarthritis Measure (JKOM). *J. Physical Med.*2008;19(4):285-90.

[33] Hirao K, Numata K, Okishima K, Tomokuni Y, Ogura T, Fujiwara K, Kobayashi R, Shimada K: Cross-sectional study of the influence of activities of daily living (ADL) on the quality of life (QOL) and daily performance in patients with symptomatic osteoarthritis of the knees. *Med. Biol.*2009;153(9):399-406.

[34] Hasegawa K: Psychology of the aged patient and the nursing approach. Kangogaku Zasshi 1974;38(8):893-900.
[35] Sheik J, Yesavage J. Geriatric Depression Scale (GDS): recent evidence and development of a shorter version. *Clin. Gerontol.* 1986;5:165-172.
[36] Salaffi F, Cavalieri F, Nolli M, Ferraccioli G. Analysis of disability in knee osteoarthritis. Relationship with age and psychological variables but not with radiographic score. *J. Rheumatol.* 1991;18(10):1581-6.
[37] Summers MN, Haley WE, Reveille JD, Alarcón GS. Radiographic assessment and psychologic variables as predictors of pain and functional impairment in osteoarthritis of the knee or hip. *Arthritis Rheum.* 1988;31(2):204-9.
[38] Kobayashi A. Gonarthrosis. Tokyo: Nankodo;1992.
[39] Huberti HH, Hayes WC. Patellofemoral contact pressures. The influence of q-angle and tendofemoral contact. *J. Bone Joint Surg. Am.* 1984;66(5):715-24.

In: Activities of Daily Living (ADL)
Editor: Scott T. Lively

ISBN: 978-1-63463-913-2

Chapter 3

The Design of Robust Real-Time Wearable Fall Detection Systems Aiming for Fall Prevention

***D. Y. C. Lie*[1,2,*]*, B. T. Nukala*[1]*, J. Jacob*[1]*, J. Tsay*[1]*, N. Shibuya*[4]*, P. E. Lie*[3]*, A. I. Rodriguez*[2]*, T. Q. Nguyen*[1,2] *and S. Zupancic*[2]**

[1]Department of Electrical and Computer Engineering, Texas Tech University (TTU), Lubbock, Texas, US
[2]Texas Tech University Health Sciences Center (TTUHSC), Lubbock, Texas, US
[3]Lubbock High School, Lubbock, Texas, US
[4]On leave from the Department Electrical and Electronic Eng., Tokushima University, Tokushima, Japan

Abstract

Falls are dangerous among the elderly population and are a major health concern. Many investigators and some commercial products have used accelerometers for real-time fall detection. Furthermore, the combination of miniature 3-D accelerometers and gyroscopes has also

---

[*] Corresponding author: D. Y. C. Lie. E-mail: Donald.Lie@ttu.edu.

been used for fall detection sensors, but the effects of the optimal placement position of these sensors have not been studied thoroughly. Besides, intelligent algorithms can be used to improve the accuracy of these wearable fall detection sensors considerably. Therefore, in this chapter, we will report two related fall detection studies that used slightly different sensor technologies and smart algorithms as follows: (1) the 1st study reports our custom-designed wired sensor (with both an accelerometer and two gyroscopes) placed as a single unit on three different positions along the thoracic vertebrae on subjects (i.e., T-4, T-7, and T-10). Results indicated that T-10 was not a good location for fall detection; however, both T-4 and T-7 were suitable, with the results for T-4 being slightly better. Using a simple rule-based multi-thresholds algorithm that utilizes the recorded resultant gravitational acceleration, angular change, angular velocity, and angular acceleration, we were able to successfully detect all 60 falls and differentiate between falls and activities of daily living (ADL) with no false positives on young volunteers (note: backward falls were not included in this sensor placement study as we were using a wired sensor). This naturally leads to our second study: (2) a real-time fall detection system using our improved *wireless* gait analysis sensor (WGAS) will be detailed. This WGAS is capable of differentiating falls vs. various Activities of Daily Living (ADL) and the Dynamic Gait Index (DGI) tests performed by young volunteers using a Back Propagation Artificial Neural Network (BP ANN) algorithm. The WGAS, which includes a tri-axial accelerometer, 2 gyroscopes, a wireless module and a Texas Instruments (TI) MSP430 microcontroller can be worn by the subjects at either T4 (at back) or on a belt-clip (in front at the center of the waist) for performing the various falls, ADL, and DGI tests. The raw gait data is wirelessly transmitted from the WGAS to a nearby PC for real-time fall classification, where six features were extracted for the BP ANN. Overall fall classification accuracies of 97.0% and 97.4% have been achieved for the data taken at the T4 and at the belt positions, respectively. The preliminary data demonstrates an overall sensitivity of 97.0% and overall specificity of 97.2% for this WGAS fall detection system, suggesting this can be a good candidate as a real-time low-cost and effective fall detection device for wireless acute-care and wireless assisted-living. We are now collecting more clinical data using the WGAS system on both patients and volunteers for gait analysis targeting for fall prevention as well.

Introduction

Falls are very common among the elderly population, which can lead to high health care costs and mortality [1-3]. After a serious fall has occurred, the fear of future falling can also tax a heavy psychological toll on the patient, leading to functional declines and may even eventually limit the elderly person to be placed in an institution [4]. Numerous researchers have performed fall detection using body-worn accelerometers [5-7]. Several accelerometer-based fall detection reports use simple threshold values to differentiate between falls and activities of daily living (ADL) for patients. These systems mostly rely on a single threshold value to detect whether an activity is considered as a fall or simply an ADL, therefore are prone to false positives. In addition, an accelerometer-only system cannot measure movements with constant velocities and is limited in its use for serious gait analysis for potential fall *prevention* for an individual patient. Similarly, research work has been conducted where gyroscopes were used to detect falls [8, 9]. This kind of more sophisticated sensor system will have more data to base on to clearly distinguish between falls and ADL using simple threshold-based algorithms, as well as providing more info on gaits. Therefore, we have used both miniaturized accelerometers and gyroscopes and placed them together for realizing a robust fall detection system. Most of the reported fall detection sensors using accelerometers have been placed near the trunk or the thigh regions [5-7], and the gyroscopes alone have usually been placed on the anterior aspect of the trunk [8, 9]. Since our interest lies on fall detection of the elderly, it is expected that one would rather have a device on their backs than on the front on their chests [10]. Commercially wearable gait analysis systems are available (e.g., SwayStar™ [11]) and can be with very high resolution (< 0.01 degree/sec). However, that kind of gait analysis system is very expensive, bulky, heavy, and not FDA-approved. We hope the wearable gait sensors and algorithms custom developed at Texas Tech University (TTU) can be used as low-cost and robust fall detection sensors for wireless acute care, and also for gait analysis and fall risk assessment for fall prevention and wireless-assisted-living.

Part (I): Fall Detection System Using TTU Wired Gait Sensor

(I.1) Sensors Basics

Finding a suitable location for the placement of both the accelerometers and gyroscopes as an integrated unit is important, as a single fall-detection sensor can be more wearable and the readings can cross-check each other to better distinguish falls vs. ADL. During our testing three places were considered as regions of interests: T-4, T-7 and T-10 in the thoracic vertebrae as shown in Figure 1. The sensors were built with commercially available components. The accelerometer used is Freescale semiconductor's MMA7341LC, which has a selectable range of +/-3g or +/-11g.

In this wired sensor work the accelerometer is set to +/-11g. The gyroscopes used are the LPR530AL dual axis gyroscope (pitch and roll) and the LY530ALH single axis gyroscope (yaw); both have a sensitivity of +/-300 °/sec and from ST Microelectronics.

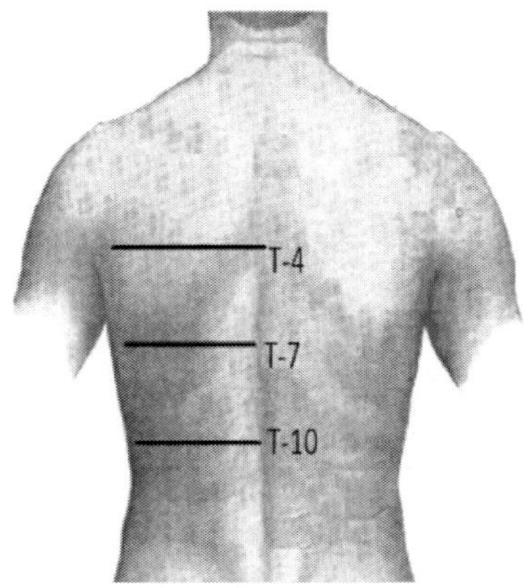

Figure 1. A view of the human thoracic vertebral column, showing regions of interest for sensor placement [12].

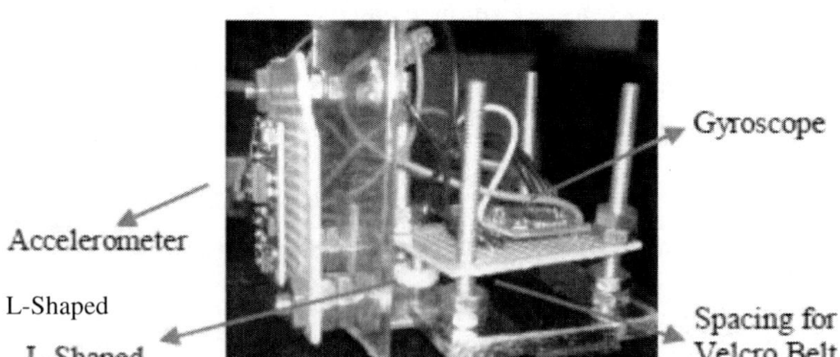

Figure 2. The device that contains the gyroscope and accelerometer sensors with a fixture used in this study. The entire device is 11 cm x 10 cm x 13 cm and weights 0.4 lb., and it can be easily mounted on a person's back.

(I.2) Methodolgy

Team members volunteered to perform the fall trials. They were asked to fall certain ways (e.g., face first, left side, right side) multiple times per condition to improve the statistical power. The same team members also performed ADL wearing the same sensors shown in Figure 2. The falls were conducted using three team members falling onto two large stacked 4" thick therapy mats. The team members ranged from 22 to 28 years of age. Each test was repeated five times. Both the gyroscope data and the accelerometer data were collected from the sensors using the National Instruments *NI-DAQ*™ USB 6009. *Matlab*™ was used as the main program for both gathering the data as well as data processing. To conduct the fall tests, data was continuously read with the *NI-DAQ*™ at a sampling rate of 1 kHz. Similarly, ADL were also recorded using the sensors shown in Figure 2. Since the main idea was to select an optimal location for the placement of the sensors for fall detection, all tests were conducted for all three regions where the sensors are placed (i.e., T-4, T-7 and T-10) and then analyzed.

(I.3) Results

Using the data recorded from the accelerometer and the gyroscopes, a simple rule-based multi-thresholds algorithm was developed to calculate the gravitational acceleration, the angular velocity and the angular acceleration (i.e., the derivative of angular velocity) recorded by the sensors. All these three parameters were calculated for all fall and ADL as shown in Figure 3. Note that during falls and ADL only the peak values are plotted here. The use of the peak values is important because sometimes the peak value may not always happen during the exact time of the fall but may be occurring slightly afterwards. For example, the accelerometer might record a high value when the subject is about to sit down but the gyroscope will record a high value when the subject is fully upright on the chair.

We have, therefore, allowed a freedom of 300ms across the peaks of the accelerometer and gyroscope data. For example if we detect a peak in the accelerometer data at 3.4 s, we will check the gyroscope data between 3.1 to 3.7 seconds to detect a peak in the gyroscope data and vice-versa.

The results from the falls and ADL are shown in Figure 3. We have recorded data from several different falls: falling forward (FF), falling sideways (FS), falling forward knee flexion (FF KF), falling sideways to the right (FSR), and falling sideways to the left (FSL). For ADL we have recorded when the subject is sitting down in a chair, when standing up, and when walking with a norm speed. Looking at the data we can clearly see that T-10 is the worst location for the sensors placement, since there is a large overlap between the highest recorded values for ADL and the lowest recorded values for falls. T-7 and T-4 regions can be used since from the recorded data we can distinguish falls from ADL; however, when we examine the highest recorded values of ADL vs. the lowest recorded values of falls, T-4 sensors data generally exhibits a slightly larger separation with better distinction. For example, the lowest recorded value of falls by the gyroscope was 2.74 rad/sec and of the highest recorded ADL was 2.5 rad/sec when sensors are placed at the T-4 region, while for the T-7 region the highest recorded value of the ADL was 2.34 rad/sec and the lowest value of falls was 2.38 rad/sec. Therefore, T-4 should be close to the optimal location when we place both the integrated 3D gyroscope with the 3D accelerometer at the back for fall detection.

From the data collected, the minimum threshold values for falls were determined for the case of T-4 placement. The equations used to calculate the resultant gravitational acceleration, angular velocity, angular acceleration and total angular change are given below.

$$ResultantGravitationalAcc. = \sqrt{A_x{}^2 + A_y{}^2 + A_z{}^2}$$

$$ResultantAngularVelocity = \sqrt{\omega_x{}^2 + \omega_y{}^2 + \omega_z{}^2}$$

$$ResultantAngularAcc. = \sqrt{(\frac{d}{dt}\omega_x)^2 + (\frac{d}{dt}\omega_y)^2 + (\frac{d}{d}(\omega_z)^2}$$

$$Total\ Angular\ Change = \sum\sqrt{x^2 + y^2 + z^2}$$

The threshold values are set as 2.73g for the accelerometer, 2.74 rad/sec for the resultant angular velocity and 0.04 rad/sec^2 for the resultant angular acceleration. Using these threshold values we were able to distinguish between falls and ADL successfully.

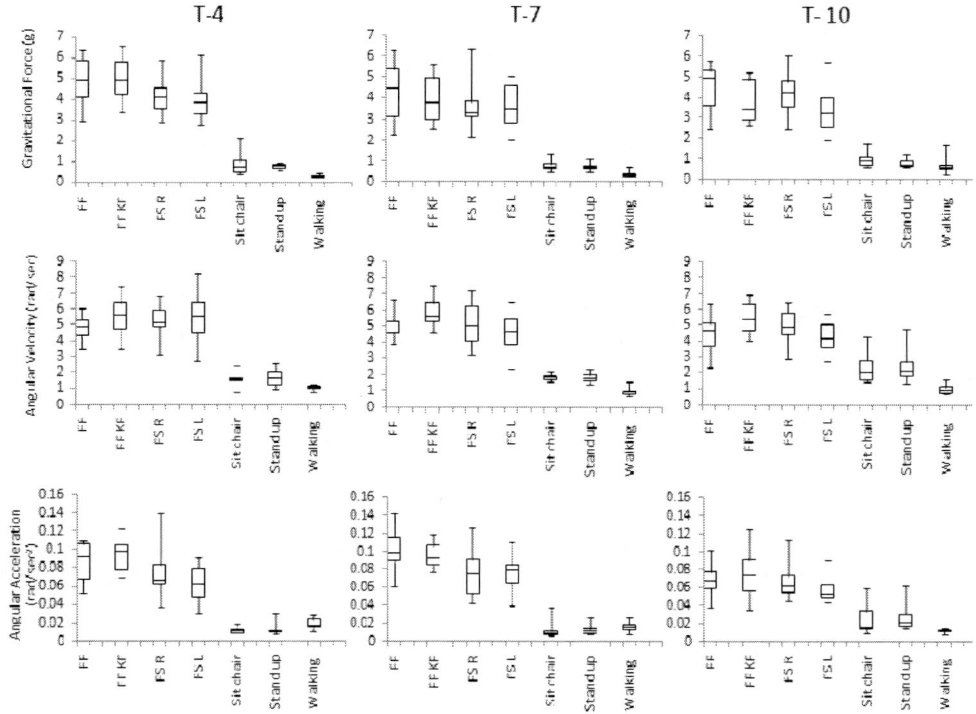

Figure 3. Box plots showing the peak values of measured acceleration, angular velocity and angular acceleration at T-4, T-7 and T-10 for different falls and ADL. FF: Falling Forward, FS: Falling Sideways, KF: Knee Flexion, R: Right, L:Left. The upper edge of each box indicates the 75th percentile of the data value and the lower edge of the box plot indicates the 25th percentile of the data value. The line inside each box indicates the median. The ends of the vertical lines indicate the maximum and the minimum values of each dataset (i.e., the data range).

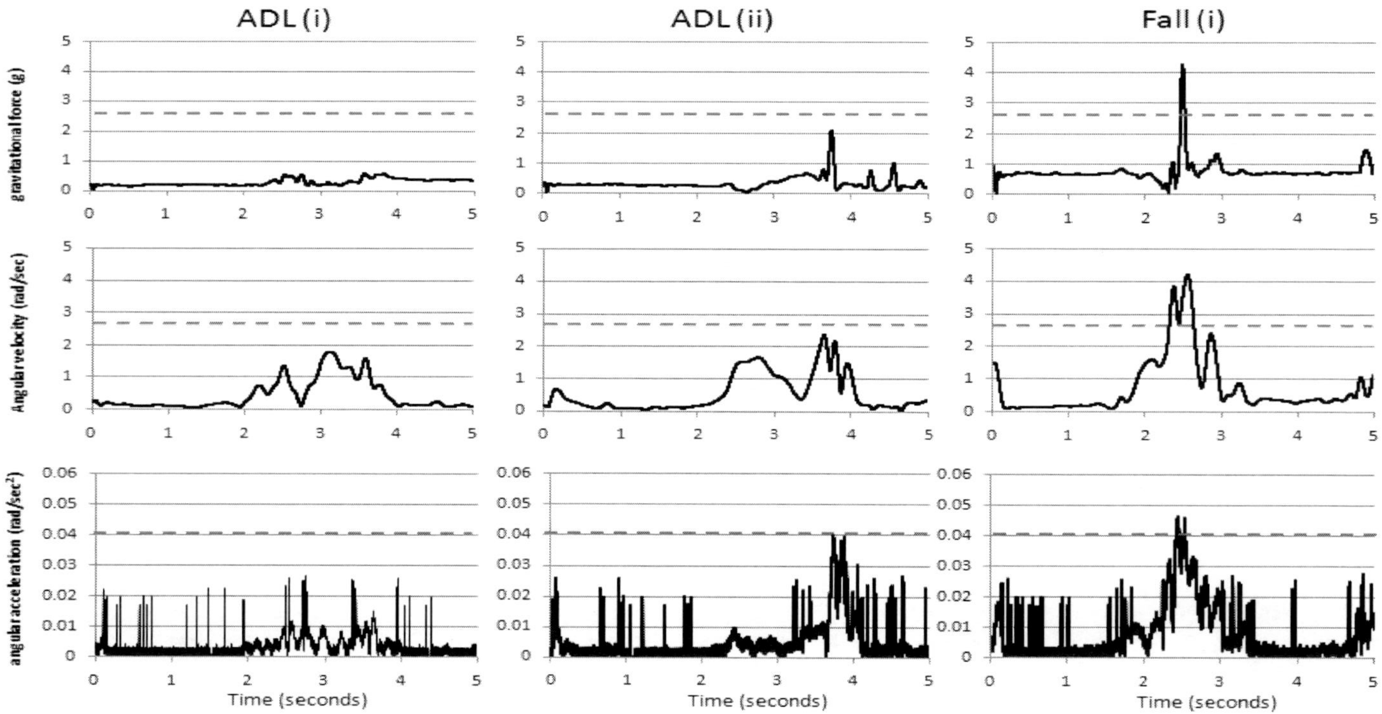

Figure 4. The resultant gravitational acceleration, angular velocity and angular acceleration from several ADL cases. (Left): ADL(i), an ADL that did not exceed any thresholds; (MIDDLE): ADL(ii): an ADL that has only the angular acceleration close to the threshold; and (RIGHT): Fall (i). Note if the sensor data exceeds all three threshold values, it will automatically be classified as a fall.

From Figure 4, one can see that the data of ADL(i) did not exceed any threshold values (red dashed lines), so it cannot be classified as a fall.

For ADL(ii) and Fall(i) shown in Figure 4, one can see that their angular acceleration are close to each other. Since we also calculate the thresholds of the resultant gravitational acceleration and the resultant angular velocity, and that ADL(ii) only has its angular acceleration close to its threshold, it cannot be classified as a fall. Note in our initial algorithm, if *all three thresholds* are exceeded, it will automatically be classified as a fall. However, after considering an actual fall case where the sensed data only exceed two threshold value but not three thresholds, we have improved our algorithm by using additional thresholds from the angular changes from the gyroscope data. Figure 5 shows a flowchart of our simple but effective thresholds-based fall detection algorithm. Note here we also used the total angular change threshold and the thresholds of each axial angular orientation (i.e., the 3 angular changes in the individual axes) in our fall detection algorithm. Here the threshold value for the resultant total angular change was set to be 31° (i.e., "Th4" in Figure 5). To detect a person falling, a threshold value of -21° in the y-axis is used (i.e., "Th6" in Figure 5). Similarly, after taking the absolute value of the data from the X-axis, a threshold value of 25°was set (i.e., "Th5" in Figure 5) and the threshold for angular change in the Z-axis was 21° (i.e., "Th7" in Figure 5). In this manner, we were able to successfully detect all falls. It needs to be noted that angular change should be used along with other thresholds from the angular acceleration and gravitational force experienced by the sensors. For example, there was one fall case where angular change did not go above any of the threshold values; however, using the entire set of the 4 threshold values, all 60 falls were successfully detected within 2 seconds with no false positives, as will be explained next. Let us look at these realistic scenarios we encountered: there is one measured fall data that has a peak value of 2.7g, below the gravitational acceleration threshold value of (2.73g); and there is a 2nd fall data that has a peak value of 2.7rad/sec, below the angular velocity threshold of 2.74rad/sec. If we consider a total of 60 falls, and calculate the fall detection sensitivity for this 1st case (Table I, 1st row), we can see that if we use the accelerometer threshold only we will miss detecting this 1st fall and achieve 98.33% sensitivity. Similarly if we use the angular velocity as the only threshold we will miss detecting the 2nd fall and achieve 98.33% sensitivity. Now if we use both the gravitational acceleration and the angular velocity thresholds, the fall detection sensitivity will drop even further because now two falls are not detected since they do not pass both of the two threshold values (i.e., sensitivity of 96.33% in Table I).

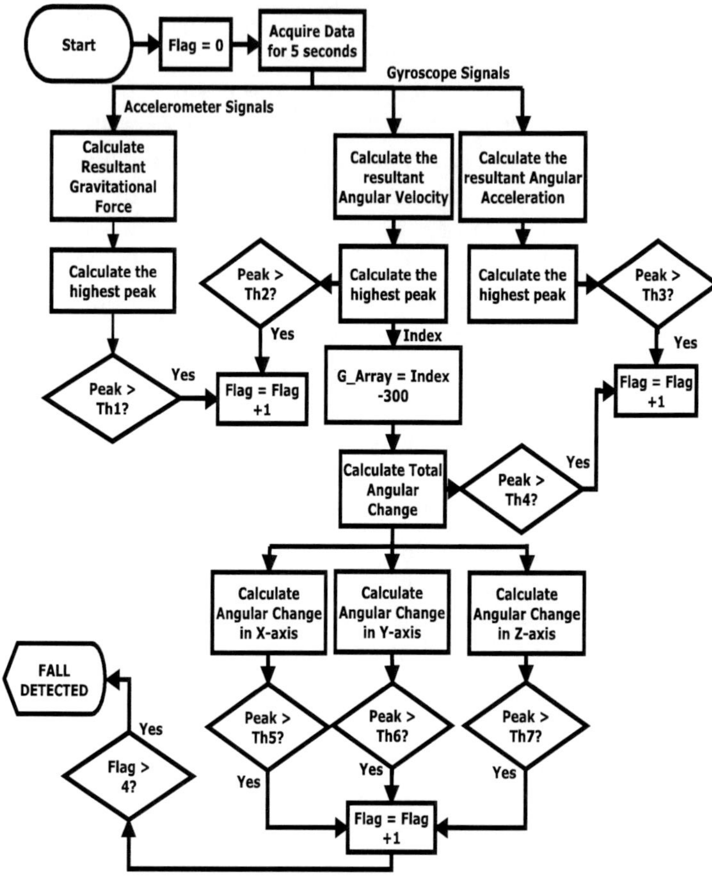

Figure 5. A flowchart of our rule-based multi-thresholds algorithm for fall detection. Th1: accelerometer threshold; Th2: angular velocity threshold; Th3: angular acceleration threshold; Th4: total angular change threshold; Th5: angular change in the X-axis threshold; Th6: angular change in the Y-axis threshold; Th7: Angular change in the Z-axis threshold.

However, if we take into accounts of the gravitational acceleration, angular velocity, angular acceleration and total angular change as the threshold values (i.e., Th1, Th2, Th3, Th4), and if we consider an event as a fall where as long as three out of the four thresholds have been exceeded, we are able to achieve 100 percent sensitivity as shown in Table 1. Similarly, if we use four out of seven threshold values, we can achieve 100 percent sensitivity as well. Using this simple algorithm that considers all 7 thresholds as shown in Figure 5, 100 percent specificity is obtained for these 60 falls.

Table 1. Fall detection sensitivity percentage obtained using our simple rule-based multi-thresholds algorithm from sensors mounted at T-4

Different Thresholds to Classify Falls	Sensitivity (%)
Accelerometer (Th1) only	98.33
Angular velocity threshold (Th2) only	98.33
Angular acceleration threshold (Th3) only	100
Two thresholds together (Th1, Th2)	96.66
Two thresholds together (Th2,Th3)	98.33
Three thresholds out of four (Th1, Th2, Th3, Th4)	100
Four thresholds out of seven (Th1, Th2, Th3, Th4, Th5, Th6, Th7)	100

More fall data is needed to improve the robustness of the threshold values selection and specificity.

(I.4) Summary and Future Work from the Wired Fall Detection Sensor Study

Placing both the 3-D accelerometers and 3-D gyroscopes in different locations on a person's back, we were able to find a suitable location for the concurrent placement of our sensors close to the T-4 region. We also developed a simple thresholds-based algorithm by calculating the gravitational force, the resultant angular velocity, the resultant angular acceleration, etc. In this manner, all 60 falls were successfully detected and with no false positives. In our fall detection algorithm we use the threshold values from the gravitational force, angular velocity and angular acceleration along with the resultant angular change and the angular change of each individual axis. If an event exceeds 4 or more threshold values, then the event will be classified as a fall. Using this simple algorithm we have accomplished a sensitivity of 100 percent with no false positives on young volunteers. Table II shows the summary of our prototype system's preliminary test results on young volunteers compared with other fall detection systems reported.

Presently, the system collects 5 seconds of data and the analysis is later done in *MatLab*™. This data analysis can be further improved by using real-time software like *LABVIEW*™ and with wireless transmission and smaller fixture size. It can also be improved by creating an adaptive algorithm along with a height and weight profile to automatically calculate the necessary threshold values for each individual.

Table 2. Summary and comparison of our system with other fall detection systems

Paper	Accelerometer	Gyroscope	Specificity (%)	Fall Dataset	Placement of sensors
[6]	2	0	100	240	Trunk and Thigh
[8]	2	2	92	70	Chest and Thigh
[9]	0	1	100	240	Sternum
[13]	1	1	96.7	60	Chest
This Work	1	2	100	60	Both on T-4 at back

Therefore, more data needs to be collected, including additional falls (especially backwards falling data that is lacking here in this work because our sensor is not wireless yet) and other activities of daily living.

Part (II): 2nd Wireless Fall Detection Study Using Our Wireless Gait Analysis Sensor (WGAS) System

(II.1) Introduction on Gait Analysis and Fall Detection

Approximately one third of the population over 65 years of age fall at least once every year, and the probability of falling increases proportionally with age. Statistics shows that 53% of senior adults who required hip surgeries related subsequent to a fall will encounter another fall within six months of being released from the hospital [14]. Along with muscle weakness and vision impairment, vestibular disorders are one of the main causes of serious falls in the geriatric population [15]. In a mid-size nursing home with 100 beds, it is estimated that one serious fall will occur every day [14], making it important to be able to wirelessly detect and record falls in both acute care and assisted living settings. For patients with dementia, the need for a robust and easy-to-use real-time automatic fall detection system is relevant as these patients often cannot recall what initiated their fall and the severity of the fall itself. Unless these risk factors are removed, patients will continue to be considered at risk for further falls and injury. Therefore, numerous methods have been proposed to perform automatic fall detection. A skin contact sensor was proposed that used the norms of the tri-axial accelerometer to detect falls [16].

A shock sensor made of a piezoelectric material and a mercury tilt switch was proposed to recognize effects and orientation of the subject [17]. Various radio tags attached to the body were utilized together with machine learning routines for fall recognition [18]. Acceleration vectors generated from the tri-axial accelerometers at trunk and thigh were used in calculating their norms for fall detection [19].

Many fall detection analysis focused around the use of threshold based techniques (i.e., if the signal exceeds the threshold(s) then a fall is detected).

However, finding the suitable threshold value(s) that can reliably detect all kinds of falls has proven to be a difficult task, and more sophisticated algorithms are needed to improve the specificity and sensitivity for real-time automatic fall detection systems.

Recently, a few companies have come up with their proprietary fall-detection systems for clinical use, such as [20]:

- *Actibelt*: uses a 3D-accelerometer hidden in a belt buckle (Trium GmbH);
- *iVi Intelligent Pendant*: can detect serious falls and send an alert (Tunstall);
- *AutoAlert system with Lifeline*: can detect falls and automatically call for help if it detects a fall (Philips);
- *PAMSys* (Biosensics): gait analysis but not real-time fall detection;
- *Shimmer3:* provides real-time inertial sensing via accelerometers, gyroscopes, magnetometers and altimeter and with an integrated motion processor for on-board 3D orientation estimation (Realtime Technologies).

We have studied fall detection using our custom sensor without the wireless feature and achieved 100% accuracy in identifying all 60 falls vs. the activities of daily living (ADL), with no false positives on young volunteers using threshold based algorithms [21].

For the current project, the sensor is wireless and allows for real-time untethered testing for not only fall detections, but also for gait analysis [21, 22]. This paper reports our new Wireless Gait Analysis Sensor (WGAS) used specifically for real-time automatic fall detection with an efficient BP ANN algorithm. This WGAS is placed and tested at two different positions on the body: at T4 and at the belt using a belt clip as shown in Figure 6. We will show the statistical data with analysis on all fall tests.

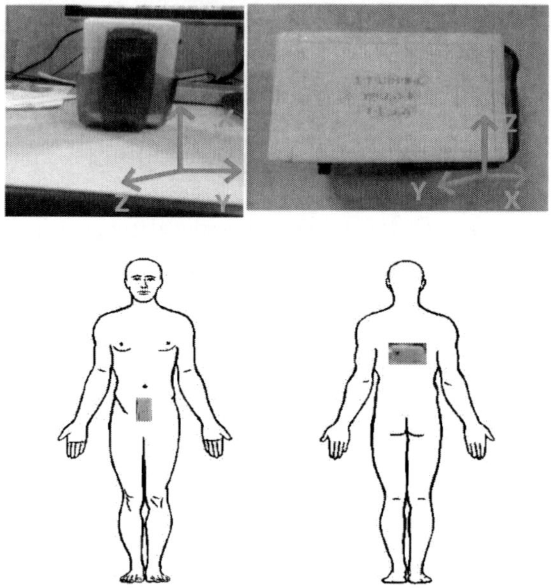

Figure 6. Sensor orientation and location on the belt-clip position (left) and at T4 (right).

(II.2) Sensor System and Experimental Methods

a. The Wireless Gait Analysis Sensor (WGAS)

The custom-designed WGAS consists of a3-axis linear accelerometer, a single axis gyroscope, and a dual axis gyroscope to measure 3-D human body translations and rotations during a gait pattern with the help of these Micro-Electrical and Mechanical system (MEMS) sensors integrated on a PCB. This WGAS system is supported by a Texas Instruments (TI) MSP430 microcontroller, and a wireless 2.4 GHz USB transceiver using the *SimpliciTI*™ protocol with a range of ~12 meters (40 ft). The 2 AAA batteries used in our earlier wired sensor [20] were replaced by a single rechargeable Li-ion coin battery, providing a battery lifetime of ~48 hours continuous operation time with each recharge. The PCB, coin battery and the microcontroller are placed in a specially designed 3D printed box $(2.2' \times 1.5' \times 0.8')$ with a total weight of 42 grams. The design of the box was done with a 3D modeling software Rhinoceros (Rhino) and printed using a 3D printer with acrylonitrile butadiene styrene (ABS) plastic. The box has a sliding lid and shown in Figure 7.

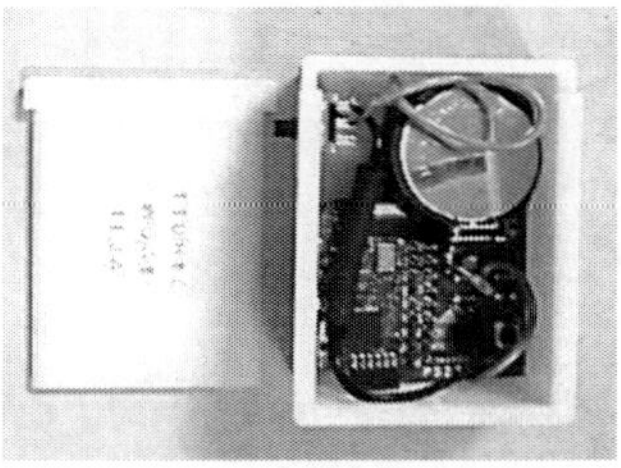

Figure 7. Physical structure of the WGAS.

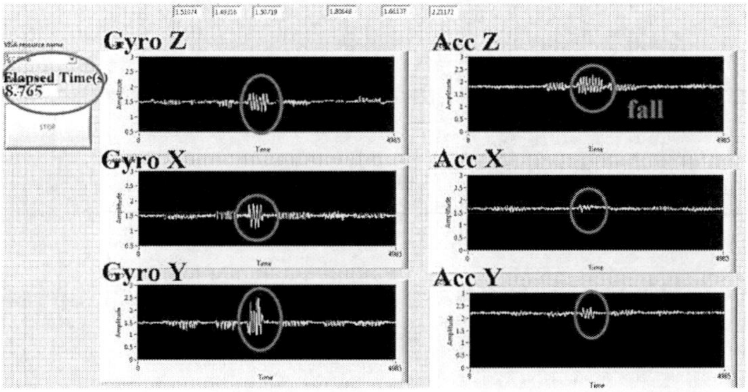

Figure 8. GUI designed *in LABVIEW™* for our real-time fall detection system using the WGAS, indicating a fall occurred after 8.765 sec.

The accelerometer data is sampled at 160 Hz and digitized to 8 bits, with its output scaled to ±6g at ($\Delta V = \pm 6g/V_{DD}\ (V_{DD} = 3.6\ V)$ for each axis. The gyroscope data is also sampled at 160 Hz and digitized to 8 bits, with its output scaled to 300° per sec. (dps) at $\Delta V = \pm 300dps/So$ (*So*(sensitivity) typical value = 3.752 mV/dps for the accelerometer and 3.33 mV/dps for the gyroscopes). The sensor orientation and positions on the body are shown in Figure 6. The sensor is carefully secured to the subjects during testing to avoid artifacts. The microcontroller and the transceiver unit enables the real-time transmission of the 6-dimensionalgait data wirelessly to the nearby PC, where a LABVIEW™ program is used for designing the Graphical User Interface (GUI) (Figure 8).

b. Testing of Fall, ADL and DGI

Intentional falls similar to those reported in [16] were performed on a gymnastics cushioned landing mat (approximately 8" thick) by two young volunteers wearing the WGAS at T4 and on the belt (see Table 3 with 10 types of falls). The total number of falls was 101 (51 at T4 and 50 at belt).

Table 3. Intentional falls performed in this work [16]

Test No.	Description
1.	Fall back with legs straight
2.	Fall forward with legs straight
3.	Fall back with knees bent
4.	Fall forward with knees bent
5.	Fall left with knees bent
6.	Fall right with knees bent
7.	Fall left with legs straight
8.	Fall right with legs straight
9.	Fall while sitting on a chair
10.	Trip over a small object

Table 4. Activities of Daily Living (ADL) movements performed [16]

Test No.	Description
1.	Sitting down and standing up from an armchair
2.	Sitting down and standing up from a low stool
3.	Sitting down and standing up from a bed
4.	Lying down and standing up from a bed
5.	Walking 10 m
6.	Stretching while standing
7.	Picking up an object from the floor

Table 5. Dynamic Gait Index (DGI) tests performed

No.	Description
1.	Gait level surface – walk with the normal speed up to 20' mark
2.	Change in Gait speed- walk with normal pace up to 5'.walk fast for next 5', walk slowly for next 5' and walk normal for last 5'
3.	Gait with horizontal head turns-walk normal with horizontal head turns up to 20' mark
4.	Gait with vertical head turns-walk normal with vertical head turns up to 20' mark
5.	Gait and Pivot turn-walk normal but at the end turn around like a pivot turn
6.	Step over obstacle-walk normal and when you come across obstacle step over not around
7.	Step around obstacles-walk normal and when 1st obstacle comes across, walk around right side and when 2nd obstacle comes across walk around left

For the ADL tests [16], the same volunteers performed every ADL recorded in Table 4 (including picking up an object test #7), and the aggregate number of ADL was 69 (34 at T4 and 35 at belt). For the DGI tests [23], the same volunteers performed every DGI test in Table 5, with 152 tests (82 at T4 and 70 at belt).

(II.3) BP ANN Algorithm

Back Propagation Artificial Neural Network (BP ANN) has been applied in numerous areas with excellent results, for example in extraction, classification and prediction [24]. In this paper six simple features (2 for each axis) were extracted from the accelerometer and gyroscope sensors for each of the falls, ADL and DGI tests, which are used as the inputs for the classification algorithm as shown in Equations 1-2:

Angular velocity Range:

$$R_{\omega,x} = \max(\omega_x) - \min(\omega_x); R_{\omega,y} = \max(\omega_y) - \min(\omega_y);$$
$$R_{\omega,z} = \max(\omega_z) - \min(\omega_z)\ldots \quad (1)$$

Acceleration Range:

$$R_{a,x} = \max(A_x) - \min(A_x);$$
$$R_{a,y} = \max(A_y) - \min(A_y); R_{a,z} = \max(A_z) - \min(A_z)\ldots \quad (2)$$

a. Back Propagation Artificial Neural Network (BP ANN)

In the training of the feed-forward ANN classifier, back propagation was applied according to Duda et al. [25]. Similar to described in [26], a 3-layer system was picked as the standard BP ANN. The input layer of the network has six neurons which correspond to the six input feature values. There is one hidden layer holding 10 hidden neurons, which number was optimized by adjusting the size of hidden neurons (from one to 15) as shown in Figure 6, where two output neurons corresponding to the two target classes the network needs to differentiate (the features of all falls are considered as class 1, and all DGI and ADL are as class 2).

The multiplication factors of the connections between the layers (or the weightings (W)) are randomly generated between -0.15 to +0.15. The training, validation and testing of the ANN classifier was performed by dividing the input feature data sets to 70%, 15% and 15% of its total, respectively.

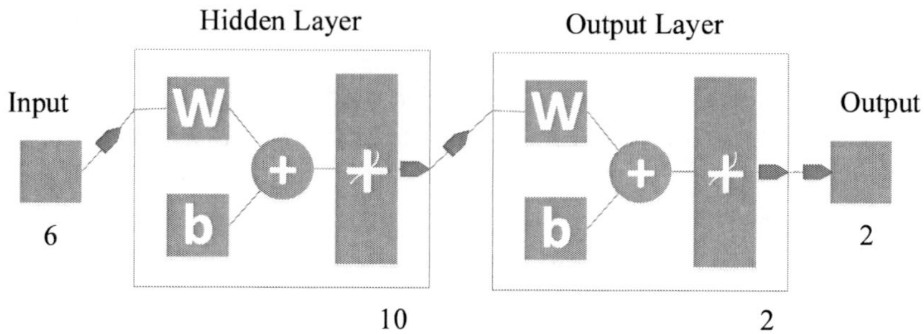

Figure 9. The 3-layer BP ANN topology used in this work.

Table 6. BP ANN classification results and final parameters from T4 data

Parameters	
Number of Input Neurons	6
Number of Hidden Neurons	10
Number of Output Neurons	2
Learning Coefficient	0.75
% of Error	3%
Number of Epochs	19
Training*	SCG
Gradient	0.0162
Training optimization time (s)	0.00
Number of training dataset	117
Number of test data set	25
Number of Validation data set	25
Training dataset CDR	96.6%
Test dataset CDR	100%
Validation dataset CDR	96.0%
Overall CDR	97.0%

*SCG = Scaled Conjugate Gradient.

The learning coefficient of the network is adjusted to 0.75 during various experiments until the cross entropy values of the training, validation and testing data sets are small enough (i.e., less than 1).

(II.4) Classification Results

Fall detection using BP ANN was done on WGAS data taken at both T4 and belt positions. The data was obtained using a 1.7 GHz PC with 4 GB of

RAM, Windows 8 OS and, and the MATLAB R2013b for the BP ANN classifier model. For the trained BP ANN classifier model, the same number of training, validation and testing datasets was used. The BP ANN classifier model learned and converged after 19 epochs for the data from T4 position. The results at T4 were obtained as follows: using the training dataset yielded 96.6% Correct Detection Rate (CDR), while using testing and validation dataset yielded 100% and 96.0% CDRs, respectively. Combining training, testing and validation detection results yielded an overall CDR of 97.0%.

The performance of the BP ANN classifier is determined by the validation cross entropy. Minimizing the cross entropy can give better results. In this case the best validation performance was achieved at epoch 13 with a cross entropy of 0.091.The performance indicators such as specificity and sensitivity were also calculated by using the Equations 3-4:

$$Specificity = \frac{TN}{TN + FP} \tag{3}$$

$$Sensitivity = \frac{TP}{TP + FN} \tag{4}$$

where *TN* (true negatives) are the ADLs and DGIs correctly classified, *FP* (false positives) are the ADLs and DGIs that were not correctly classified by the BP ANN, *TP* (true positives) are the falls correctly classified and *FN* (false negatives) are the falls that were not detected by the BP ANN. The specificity of the BP ANN for fall detection at T4 is 96.5% and the sensitivity is 98.0%.

Figure 10 shows the box plots for the ADLs vs. falls listed in Table 3 and Table 4taken at T4. The maximum ranges were recorded for Gyro X (for ADL 4 and ADL 7: 0.81V and 0.69V, respectively), and Acc Y (for ADL 4 and ADL 7:0.30V and 0.19V, respectively). For the falls, the maximum ranges were recorded for the Gyro X (for Fall 2 and Fall 9: 1.13V and 1.02V, respectively) and Acc Y (for fall 10 and fall 9: 0.66V and 0.59V, respectively). Some more statistics are shown in Table 7 for the T4 data.

The BP ANN classifier model learned and converged after 12 epochs for the data taken at the belt position.

The results at the belt position were obtained as follows: using the training dataset yielded 98.2% CDR, while using testing and validation dataset yielded 100% and 91.3% CDRs, respectively. Combining training, testing and validation detection results yielded an overall CDR of 97.4%, similar to the values obtained for the data taken at T4.

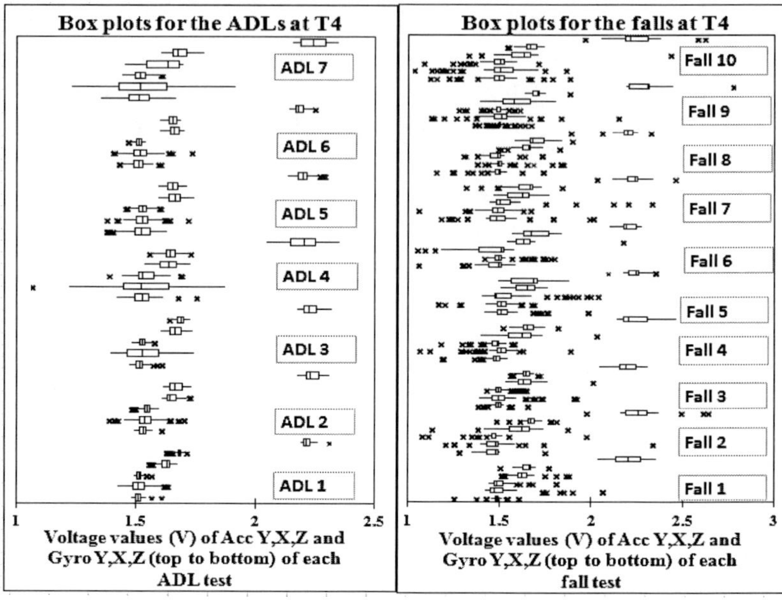

Figure 10. Box plots for the ADLs and falls listed in Tables 1-2 taken at T4.

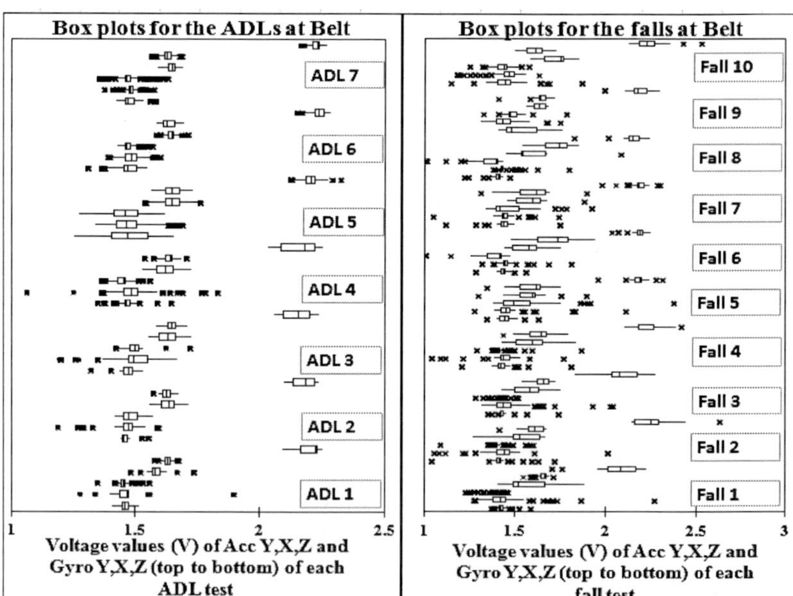

Figure 11. Box plots for the ADLs and falls listed in Tables 1-2 taken at belt.

Table 7. Statistical table for ADLs vs. falls at T4

Stats	Gyro X (ADL 4)	Acc Y (ADL 4)	Gyro X (fall 2)	Acc Y (fall 10)
Mean	1.532	2.201	1.482	2.234
STDEV	0.134	0.071	0.153	0.101
Min.	1.062	2.050	1.206	1.956
Median	1.522	2.205	1.479	2.208
Max.	1.871	2.352	2.331	2.616
Range	0.81	0.302	1.125	0.66

Table 8. Statistical table for ADLs vs. falls at belt

Stats	Gyro X (ADL 4)	Acc Y (ADL 4)	Gyro X (fall 2)	Acc X (fall 7)
Mean	1.495	2.151	1.431	1.591
STDEV	0.088	0.068	0.114	0.093
Min.	1.059	2.033	1.044	1.306
Median	1.487	2.179	1.446	1.617
Max.	1.830	2.246	2.008	1.892
Range	0.77	0.213	0.964	0.586

Figure 11 shows the box plots for ADLs vs. falls taken at belt. The maximum ranges were recorded for Gyro X (for ADL 4 and ADL 1: 077V/ 0.6V, respectively) and Acc Y (for ADL 4 and ADL 3:0.21V/0.17V, respectively). For falls, the maximum ranges were recorded for Gyro X (for Fall 2 and Fall 1: 0.96V/0.92V, respectively) and Acc X (for Fall 7:0.59V), as shown in Table 6. The specificity of the BP ANN for falls detection at belt is 98.1% and sensitivity is 96.0%. In this case the best validation performance was achieved at epoch 6 with a cross entropy of 0.283.

Table 10 shows the results of this work compared with previously published work in the literature. Please note we did not include [16] in Table 8 because the testing subjects for falls vs. ADL were not from the same group.

Many reported studies [19, 24, 28] uses a single 3-axial accelerometer to detect falls; also threshold based algorithms proved to be complicated yet they can be successful for fall detection.

Our WGAS uses both accelerometer and gyroscopes for real-time analysis of falls by using BP ANN algorithm is robust in detecting falls with high accuracy and sensitivity in < 0.01s.

Table 9. BP ANN classification results and final parameters (data at belt)

Parameters	
Number of Input Neurons	6
Number of Hidden Neurons Number of Output Neurons	10 2
Learning Coefficient	0.75
% of Error	2.6%
Number of Epochs	12
Training* Gradient	SCG 0.0109
Training optimization time (s)	0.00
Number of training dataset	109
Number of test dataset Number of Validation data set	23 23
Training dataset CDR	98.2%
Test dataset CDR Validation dataset CDR	100% 91.3%
Overall CDR	97.4%

*SCG = Scaled Conjugate Gradient.

Table 10. TTU real-time WGAS fall-detection system performance vs. the literature

	Sensors	Sensitivity	Specificity
[14]	1 Acc, 2 Gyro	91.0	92.0%
[15]	1 Acc	80.0%	88.0%
[6]	1 Acc	94.0%	94.0%
[11]	1 Acc	98.4%	98.6%
This work	1 Acc., 2 Gyro	98.0% (at T4) 96.0% (at belt)	96.5% (at T4) 98.1% (at belt)

Moreover, the BP ANN algorithm can also be implemented in *LABVIEW*™ next to streamline and speed up real time detection.

(II.5) Summary of WGAS Fall Detection Sensor

Our custom wireless gait analysis sensor (WGAS) was applied for real-time automatic fall detection with a simple but very fast ANN with 6 input features trained by back propagation.

The results show that falls are automatically detected at both T4 and belt positions with an overall sensitivity of 97.0% and specificity of 97.2% (i.e., 98 out of 101 falls correctly classified at both positions and 215 out of 221 ADL+DGI tests correctly classified).

The preliminary data on young volunteers suggests our real-time fall detection system performs competitively compared to other systems, whether placed at T4 or on a waist-level belt. For example, Table 10 shows the best accuracy of ~98.5% was reported in [11]; however in that work various types of falls were *not* tested so its actual specificity is expected to be lower.

Conclusion

The real-time fall detection study shown in Part (I) of this chapter uses our earlier developed wired accelerometer-gyroscope sensor with threshold-based algorithms, and the work described in Part (II) using our latest wireless gait analysis sensor (WGAS) with BP ANN; both sensors achieved excellent accuracies of fall detection rate of over 97% on volunteers.

Please note that younger subjects were used in the work presented here as proxies for older persons, which is an initial study limitation before clinical trials on actual patients. We believe that for the falls that exhibit only small acceleration, sensitive gyroscopes that can pick up noticeable angular changes are needed to detect these falls (e.g., the problematic slow falling from a chair such as fall #9 listed in Table 5).

Therefore, our fall detection systems using both accelerometers and gyroscopes can be superior to sensors using accelerometers only. Further improvement on our classifiers design and performance are also underway to better our WGAS-based fall detection system, as we are exploring the more advanced classifier such as Support Vector Machine (SVM).

Since the data collected on young volunteers has demonstrated our sensors and algorithms are effective and robust, we have just started conducting testing on patients with balance disorders as a more appropriate cohort with our WGAS system.

Future work includes conducting more fall and ADL tests on geriatric and high-risk patients to improve clinical usage of this fall detection system based on our WGAS described in Part (II), and also in parallel for fall prevention efforts conduct gait analysis on patients with balance disorders (IRB already in-place and currently going through clinical trials now).

The preliminary data on 1 patient so far looks rather promising, as in that case the WGAS system can successfully differentiate the normal vs. patients effectively. The pertinent results will be reported later in our follow-up publications.

Acknowledgments

The authors would like to sincerely thank our team members for their kind support of performing falls and other tasks. The authors are also indebted to the funding support and guidance from Mr. Shekar Rao of the Center of Innovation (Arlington, TX), Texas Instruments (TI), and the generous donation of the Keh-Shew Lu Regents Endowment Fund at the Texas Tech University.

References

[1] M. E. Tinetti, M. Speechley and S. F. Ginter, "Risk factors for falls among elderly persons living in the community," *N. Eng. J. Med.*, vol. 319, pp. 1701-1707, 1988.

[2] J. Askham, E. Glucksman, P. Owens, C. Swift, A. Tinker, and G. Yu, "Home and leisure accident research: A review of research on falls among elderly people," *International Journal of Geriatric Psychiatry*, Vol. 6, Issue 11, Pg. 825, 1990.

[3] Centers for Disease Control and Prevention, National Center for Injury Prevention and Control. *Web–based Injury Statistics Query and Reporting System (WISQARS)* [online]. Accessed December 30, 2010.

[4] B. J. Vellas, S. J. Wayne, L. J. Romero, R. N. Baumgartner, and P. J. Garry, "Fear of falling and restriction of mobility in elderly fallers," *Age and Ageing* 1997;26:189-193.

[5] N. Noury, P. Barralon, G. Virone, P. Boissy, M. Hamel, and P. Rumeau, "A smart sensor based on rules and its evaluation in daily routines," *Proc. 25th Annual Int'l Conf. of IEEE EMBS*, pp. 3286-3289, Sept. 2003.

[6] K. Bourke, J. V. O'Brien, G. M. Lyons, "Evaluation of a threshold-based tri-axial accelerometer fall detection algorithm," *Gait and Posture*, 26:194-199, 2007.

[7] Najafi, K. Aminian, A. Paraschiv-Ionescu, F. Loew, C. J. Büla, and P. Robert, "Ambulatory system for human motion analysis using a kinematic sensor: monitoring of daily physical activity in the elderly," *IEEE Trans. Biomed. Eng.*, 2003; 50: 711-23.

[8] Q. Li, J. A. Stankovic, M. A. Hanson, A. T. Barth, J. Lach, and G. Zhou, "Accurate, Fast Fall Detection Using Gyroscopes and Accelerometer-Derived Posture Information," *Proc. Sixth Int'l Workshop on Wearable and Implantable Body Sensor Networks*, p. 138-143, June 03-05, 2009.

[9] K. Bourke and G. M. Lyons, "A threshold-based fall-detection algorithm using a bi-axial gyroscope sensor" *Med. Eng. Phys.*, 30:84-90, 2008.

[10] G. Wu. "Distinguishing fall activities from normal activities by velocity characteristics," *J. Biomech.* 2000;33(11):1497-500.

[11] Balance International Innovations "SwayStar^{TM}" 15th Sept. 2010. http:// www.b2i.info/web/index.htm.

[12] Henry, Gray. Surface anatomy of the back. 1918. *Gray's Anatomy of the Human Body*, Pg. 1303. Lea and Febiger Philadelphia.

[13] J. Y. Hwang, J. M. Kang, Y. W. Jang, and H. C. Kim, "Development of Novel Algorithm and Real-time monitoring Ambulatory system using Bluetooth module for fall detection in the elderly," *Proc. 26th Annual Int'l Conf. of IEEE-EMBS,* Sept. 1-5, 2004.

[14] Centers for Disease Control and Prevention, http://www.cdc.gov/ homeandrecreationalsafety/falls/adultfalls.html.

[15] G. F. Fuller, "Falls in the elderly," *American Family Physician*, vol. 61, no. 7, pp. 2159-68, 2173-4, Apr. 1, 2000.

[16] Ravi Narasimhan, "Skin-contact sensor for automatic fall detection," *Proc. IEEE Int'lEMBS Conf.*, pp. 4038-41, 2012.

[17] G. Williams, K. Doughty, K. Cameron, and D. A. Bradley, "A smart fall and activity monitor for telecare applications," *Proc. 20th Annual Int'l Conf. of IEEE EMBS,* pp. 1151-57, 1998.

[18] M. Lustrek and B. Kaluza, "Fall detection and activity recognition with machine learning," *Informatica*, 33, 3, pp. 205-212, 2009.

[19] K. Bourke, P. van de Ven, M. Gamble, R. O'Connor, K. Murphy, E. Bogan, E. McQuade, P. Finucane, G. Olaighin, J. Nelson, "Evaluation of waist-mounted tri-axial accelerometer based fall-detection algorithms during scripted and continuous unscripted activities," *J. of Biomechanics*. Vol. 43, pp. 3051-57, 2010.

[20] S. Patel, A. Puiatti, J. Niemi, L. Williamson, A. Nelson, R. Roubenoff, J. Goldhahn, and P. Bonato, "Assessing Fall-Detection Technology for

Use in Clinical Trials," *Abs. 7th World Congress of Biomechanics*, Boston, July 6-11, 2014.

[21] J. Jacob, T. Nguyen, S. Zupancic, and D. Y. C. Lie, "A Fall Detection Study on the Sensor Placement Locations and the Development of a Threshold-Based Algorithm Using Both Accelerometer and Gyroscope," *Proc. IEEE Int'l Conf. on Fuzzy Logics*, pp. 666-671, 2011.

[22] B. T. Nukala, A. I. Rodriguez, J. Tsay, T. Hall, T. Q. Nguyen, S. Zupancic, and D. Y. C. Lie, "Evaluating Optimal Placement of Real-Time Wireless Gait Analysis Sensor with Dynamic Gait Index (DGI)," *Actas. IEEE Conf. on Information Systems and Techno. (CISTI)*, pp. 160-161, 2014.

[23] K. L. Perrel, A. Nelson, R. L. Goldman, S. L. Luther, N. Prieto-Lewis, and L. Z. Rubenstein, "Fall risk assessment measures: an analytic review," *J. Gerontology Series A – Biological Sciences and Medical Sciences* 56 (12): M761-766. 2001.

[24] M. Vallejo, C. V. Isaza and J. D. Lopez, "Artificial Neural Networks as an alternative to traditional fall detection methods," *Proc. 35th Annual Int'l Conf. of IEEE EMBS*, pp. 1648-51, 2013.

[25] R. O. Duda, P. E. Hart and D. G. Stork, *Pattern Classification,* New York: Wiley–Interscience; 2001.

[26] S. Dreiseitl and L. Ohno-Machado, "Logistic regression and artificial neural network classification models: a methodology review," *J. Biomed. Inform.*, 35:352-9 2002.

[27] Q. Li, J. A. Stankovic, M. A. Hanson, A. T. Barth, J. Lach, and G. Zhou," Accurate, fast fall detection using gyroscopes and accelerometer-derived posture information," *Proc. IEEE 6th Int'l Workshop on Wearable and Implantable Body Sensor Networks (BSN)*, pp. 138-143. 2009.

[28] J. T. Perry, S. Kellog, S. M. Vaidya, Y. Jong-Hoon, H. Ali, and H. Sharif, "Survey and evaluation of real-time fall detection approaches," *Proc. IEEE 6th Int'l Symp. on High-Capacity Optical Networks and Enabling Technologies (HONET)*, pp. 158-64, 2009.

In: Activities of Daily Living (ADL)
Editor: Scott T. Lively
ISBN: 978-1-63463-913-2

Chapter 4

Disability and Ethnicities

***Elva Dolores Arias-Merino*[1,•], *Carlos Arturo González-Núñez*[2], *Neyda Ma. Mendoza-Ruvalcaba*[3] *and Beatriz A. Corona-Figueroa*[1]**

[1]Centro Universitario de Ciencias de la Salud, Universidad de Guadalajara. Edificio N. Col. Independencia, Guadalajara, Jalisco, México

[2]Centro Universitario de los Altos, Universidad de Guadalajara, México

[3]Centro Universitario de Tonalá, Universidad de Guadalajara, México

Abstract

Disability in the elderly is a complex, dynamic and multidimensional condition. Recently, there has been a shift from an exclusively individual and medical perspective of disability to a new perspective which includes social-cultural factors. There is an interrelation between disability and functionality very similar to those that exist between health and disease. Disability has been linked to frailty, cognitive decline, higher prevalence

[•] E-mail: elvadolores@yahoo.com.

of comorbidities, hospitalizations, mortality; impact in family life, stress, high costs, and health attention needs due to the increasing population of elderly. The WHO World Health Survey 2002-2004 reported a general worldwide prevalence of 38.1% in population 60 years or older, being higher in people of lower income countries, in women and in people who live in rural areas. Evaluation of disability is based on scales that report limitations of activities of daily living (ADL); these activities are divided into three sections: basic ADL, instrumental or intermediate ADL, and advanced ADLs. These instruments are widely used in diagnosing disability and in evaluating successful aging. However, there can be a great bias (if not corrected) that could influence the interpretation of its results: education and cultural differences. Activities of daily living are measured in a subjective way were the elderly usually self-report their results. Cultural differences influence in variation of results since activities of daily living are influenced by personal, family, and social perspective. Due to this self-report, some aged people may not inform the severity of their disability. An example of this issue is demonstrated in a prospective 6 year cohort study using the sample from the 1998 Health and Retirement Study studied how cultural and ethnic factors could affect the outcome of diagnosis in activities of daily living disability. Hispanics reported lower rates of walking disability even though higher frequencies of lower-extremity dysfunction were reported.

Another example could be a study that reported institutionalization due to limitations in ADLs in the Asian American elderly, where a smaller prevalence of institutionalization in Asian elderly was found compared to non-Hispanic white elderly. This result could be explained by the cultural difference that exists in the Asian elderly population. Asians are more collective than individualists, in other words, they prefer to seek help with family members instead of assisting for help in a nursing home. In conclusion, diagnosing disability is highly influenced by cultural differences. Lack of early diagnosis could in the end, affect prevalence of frailty, cognitive decline, comorbidities, and mortality in the elderly.

Introduction

Aging of our population has caused certain concern in public health because of the social, political, and economic impact that is expected upon this phenomenon. Aging implies high costs derived from frailty, disability, and death. From an individual point of view, the biologic process of aging normally affects systems and functions of the body probably associated to chronic degenerative diseases and lifestyle behaviors leading to a gradual descent in functionality and abilities to perform activities of daily living (ADLs). This inability to perform ADLs could lead to functional impairment, disability, and in the end, death. Since 2001, the WHO proposed a new framework stressing a different point of view based on health and functioning rather than on disability. Previously, disability was believed to be a separate entity from health deterioration, producing two separate categories. It is now known that with health deterioration, an individual could experience some sort of disability; this idea has defined disability as a multidisciplinary and complex model [1].

According to this model, the term function refers to all body functions, activities and participation, while disability is viewed as an umbrella term for functional impairment, activity limitations and social participation restrictions. The Disablement Process compasses both lifelong and late-life disability [2]. To further clarify the natural history of disability, certain theories and models have been created to explain how disability is associated with life expectancy. The theories that represent the disablement process are:

- Theory of morbidity expansion: [3] this theory emphasizes on how longer life expectancy on older adults is due to technological advances and adequate preventive strategies. This longer life expectancy has also affected older adults with disability and subjacent diseases. The elderly live with non-mortal diseases like vision loss, osteoarthritis, chronic pain, among other; this implies that living more means living more years with disability.
- Theory of morbidity compression: [4, 5] Preventive strategies modify mortality risk factors, therefore provoking a delay in age of onset for disability or diseases causing disability. If life expectancy would have a maximum limit than those with disability will present it at a shorter frame, compressed by the age limit.
- Theory of Dynamic Equilibrium: [6] This theory proposes that the sum of economy, medicine, and technology have reduced mortality influencing morbidity and disability. With a reduction of mortality there is also a reduction in the incidence and progression of chronic diseases. This reduction results in an older population in the future, ending up fragile and with a higher risk for disability.
- These 3 theories form a cycle, where each theory compensates each other creating a cycle with constant movement [7].
- Medical Model on Disability: views disability as a feature in a person, directly caused by disease, trauma or other health conditions, which

require medical care provided in the form of individual treatment by health professionals.

- Social Model on Disability: sees disability as a socially-created problem and not at all an attribute of an individual. Disability demands a political response, since the problem is created by an unaccommodating physical environment brought about by attitudes and other features of the social environment.

Disability is a multidimensional phenomenon that is both a problem at the level of a person's body, and a complex and primarily social phenomenon [1]. Implies an interaction between an individual and the overall context in which the person lives. It is considered an outcome of interactions between health conditions (diseases, disorders and injuries) and contextual factors (external environmental, such as social attitudes, architectural characteristics, legal characteristics, social structures, and so forth; internal personal factors such as gender, age, copying styles, social background, education, behavior, personality and others).

Some aspects of disability are almost entirely internal to the person, while other aspects are almost entirely external; disability involves dysfunction at one or more levels which are:

- Impairment in body function or structure, including physical and mental functions.
- Activity limitations to execute a task or actions, such as self-care, mobility, domestic life, and communication.
- Participation restrictions or problems in involvement in life and social situations, as interpersonal interactions and relationships, community, social and civic life.

Disability in the elderly is even a more complex dynamic medical and social condition, where 59 out of the 70 countries included in the World Health Organization report were suffering from this condition, there is a prevalence of 38.1% worldwide in the population 60 years or older [8].

Disability has been linked to a higher risk for frailty, cognitive decline, and higher prevalence of comorbidities, hospitalizations, and mortality [9-12].

In addition, several investigations have been devoted to isolate risk factors for disability in the elderly.

Studies indicate that socio-demographic factors like age [13-15], gender, specifically being woman [13, 15], low education level [13], income or socioeconomic status [15, 16], marital status [15, 14], race [16], and being a lifelong housewife [13], are high-risk factors.

Health conditions have also been reported as important risk factors for disability, for instance, previous history of disability [13, 14], having at least one chronic disease [13], chronic disability and multi-morbidity [17], inadequate control of chronic conditions, unnecessary use of psychoactive drugs, inactivity [15], joint stiffness [18, 19], obesity [20], foot problems, heart problems, vision [19], and sarcopenia which has been associated with functional decline over a 2-year period [21].

Depression and depressive symptoms are also risk factors to be considered among other risk factors like [22, 23, 13, 16], cognitive impairment [12, 13, 19], poor health perception [14], dietary pattern [24], and even death wishes [25], have been found as psychological/behavioral risk factors strongly associated with functional disability.

Little social support [14], and social isolation are also factors that could increase the odds for disability [15].

We have described several risk factors that participate in the presentation of disability, although we believe that cultural and racial differences also play a role in the process of disability, especially in countries with diverse ethnic groups, like the United States of America and recently in the European Union, where immigration has increased throughout the years. According to the NIDR Long Range Plan (2005-2009), disability as a product of an interaction between factors that may differ between certain ethnic groups.

Currently, the identification of disability is based on limitations of activities of daily living (ADL), these activities are divided into three sections: basic ADL, instrumental or intermediate ADL, and advanced ADLs. The basic ADL consist of self-care activities that consist of bathing, eating, toileting, dressing, maintaining continence, and transferring. Once the elderly have difficulty to perform these activities they may usually end up having caregiver assistance, this could imply social and economic implications for both the elderly and their family. Instrumental ADL consist of higher-level activities which include using the telephone, shopping, doing housework, preparing meals, driving, taking medications, and managing money. The advanced ADLs are tasks that are usually affected by social integration, examples of these activities include occupational, recreational, and travel activities, these are usually characterized by personality; giving these activities an effect of a "functional signature" [26].

Activities of daily living are measured in a subjective way were the elderly usually self-report their results. It is no surprise that cultural differences could in the end provoke variation of results since activities of daily living are influenced by society, family, and personal perspective.

Hispanic Culture

It is interesting how different cultures may vary in their concept of older age and their perspective of it. These different ethnic cultures could affect certain public health issues, like disability, were some racial cultures will have a higher likelihood of risk factors and in presenting the disease. An example of this is the Hispanic population, which is one of the biggest minorities in the United States. The frequency of functional limitation, ADL limitation, or disability in this population, as shown on table 1, may vary but is usually consistent with the African American population. ADL limitations in this minority implicate certain cultural differences when compared to other ethnic groups; in fact even between the Hispanic culture there are differences, for example those who are English speakers versus Non-English speakers. An example of this difference could be explained by the 6 year prospective cohort study using the sample from the 1998 Health and Retirement Study, those who spoke Spanish had a higher prevalence for upper and lower body dysfunction when compared to Hispanics who spoke English (Table 1).

This study demonstrated how cultural and ethnic could affect the outcome of diagnosing disability. The authors in this study divided the Hispanic population between those who only spoke Spanish and those who could speak English. During this study, a self-report survey was answered, along with certain dysfunctions that were measured in this population. Although in the end the same ethnic group was being compared, there were certain differences in the results that were observed between English speakers versus Non-English speakers.

Spanish speakers complained that their primary ADL limitation was dressing versus English speakers who complained primarily on walking [27]. This self-reported ADL limitation seems quite interesting, since the same study observed a higher frequency of lower extremity dysfunction in Spanish speakers. Although the self-reported survey could present bias since some older adults may not be aware of their real dysfunctions; these dysfunctions could be partially affected by cultural factors.

Table 1. Compilation of studies depicting the Frequency of Disability, Functional Limitation or ADL limitations

Author	Population	Type of Study	Prevalence or Incidence	Characteristics/ Observations
Manasi A. Tirodkar (2008)	Hispanic Spanish Speaking (HS), Hispanic English Speaking (HE), African American (AA), Whites (W)	Prospective Cohort	Lower extremity limitations HS (27.53%) HE(15.22%) AA (17.65%) W (11.52%)	
			Upper extremity limitations HS (13.87%) HE (10.81%) AA (13.12%) W (8.79%)	
Esme Fuller-Thomson (2012)	Whites (W), Chinese (Ch) Pacific Islander (PI) Vietnamese (V), Korean (K), Japanese (J) Filipino (F), Asian Indian (AI)	Cross-Sectional	Not Institutionalized W(76.2%) Ch (86.8%) PI (88.6%) V (94.5%) K (81.2%) J (83.6%) F (90.8%) AI (95.3%)	All the participants had ADL limitations.
			Institutionalized W(23.8%) Ch (13.2%) PI (11.4%) V (5.5%) K (18.8%) J (16.4%) F (9.2%) AI (4.7%)	
Vivian C. Shih (2005)	African American (AA), Hispanic (H), White (W)	Prospective Cohort	With Physical limitations AA (74.52%), H (64.99%), W (62.66%)	Unadjusted OR for ADL limitation AA 1.58 (1.23-2.03) H 1.40 (0.89-2.20) W (Reference) Adjusted OR for Physical Limitations AA 3.20 (1.53-6.66) H 3.12 (0.95-10.28) W 2.58 (1.80-3.68)
Dorothy D. Dunlop (2005)	African American (AA), Hispanic (H), White (W)	Prospective Cohort	Functional Decline AA (18.67%), H (18.04%), W (12.89%)	Population with arthritis

Table 1. Compilation of studies depicting the Frequency of Disability, Functional Limitation or ADL limitations (Continued)

Author	Population	Type of Study	Prevalence or Incidence	Characteristics/ Observations
Tomata Y (2014)	Japanese	Prospective Cohort	16.60%	Japanese diet patterns have a protective effect against functional disability 0.77 (0.68-0.80)
Rafael Samper-Ternent (2012)	Mexican American Women (MAW) White Women (WW) Mexican American Men (MAM) White Men (WM)	Cross-Sectional	ADL disability MAW (56.5%) WW (69%) MAM (47.4%) WM (58.1%)	
			IADL disability MAW (93.3%) WW (88.1%) MAM (79.9%) WM (95.7%)	
Richard F. Hamman (1999)	Hispanics and White	Cross-Sectional	Any disability Hispanic: 63.5% White: 63.1%	Population bases in Rural Area
Esme Fuller-Thomson (2011)	Whites (W), Chinese (Ch) Pacific Islander (PI) Vietnamese (V), Korean (K), Japanese (J) Filipino (F), Asian Indian (AI)	Cross-Sectional	Functional Decline W (25.4%), PI (26.3%) V (21.6%) K (16.4%) J (17.9%) F (19.1%) AI (18.3%) Ch (17.2%)	OR for Functional Decline W 1.58 (1.49-1.68) PI 2.09 (1.73-2.54) V 1.55 (1.39-1.72) K 1.08 (0.95-1.21) J 0.86 (0.77-0.97) F 1.23 (1.13-1.35) AI 1.35 (1.22-1.50)
			ADL limitation W (9%) PI (11.4%) V (8.4%) K (6.2%) J (6.1%) F (6.3%) AI (5.8%) Ch (6.8%)	ADL limitation W 1.24 (1.13-1.36) PI 2.27 (1.73-2.97) V 1.55 (1.32-1.81) K 1.09 (0.91-1.31) J 0.69 (0.58-0.81) F 1.00 (0.87-1.15) AI 1.15 (0.98-1.36)

One of these cultural implications is the high family bond that exists in this culture. Spanish speakers trend to live more often with other family members who in the end could end up assisting them with certain limitations like walking. By receiving household assistance, the Spanish speaking Hispanics may not perceive that they have difficulty in walking [27]. Hispanic culture is usually based on family support [28]. Most elderly live with their family, affecting their perception in performing ADLs.

One of the highest risk factors observed for disability in the Hispanic elderly is a poor socioeconomic status [26, 29].This could explain why most of the elderly end up living with their families. Most Hispanics usually rely on informal jobs, leading to no opportunities for future pensions, only 40% of Mexicans rely on a pension as a source of an income, forcing them to work in informal jobs for longer periods of time [30]. These informal jobs are like a ticking bomb, the elderly at some point will have to retire with no pension, leaving them without an income to subside in their life. This problem could cause the elderly to depend on other household members [9] as a major source of income, which could be a low source of income if the household member also depends on an informal job, elevating the risk for disability. This is vicious cycle that the Hispanic elderly face in Latin America and in the United States of America, where most reside as immigrants with their families.

In the cross-sectional study, SABE, conducted in Guadalajara, Mexico, it was observed that 25.5% of the older adults in that population live with at least one family member, explaining, once again, how family support is an important factor contributing economic and social support for the Hispanic elderly [31]. This situation leads the elderly to a poor pension and difficulty in receiving proper medical attention. Another factor to be taken into account is obesity and poor adherence to medical therapy. Obesity can lead in the end to disability; this problem has been observed to have a higher rate among Mexican Americans when compared to Caucasians [32]. Hispanics are more likely to have chronic comorbid conditions, like hypertension, although most won't usually adhere to the medical treatment, exercise, and diet programs [33], leading to increasing risk for disability [30, 34]. Probably the low social economic status and language as a barrier in this population could explain why Hispanics are at higher risk for ADL limitations. Poor understanding of their disability and high rate of family help for their disability could slowdown institutional help.

Disability is not only more prevalent in the Hispanic urban community, compared to Caucasians; this is also observed in rural communities [35]. The constant factors that this population faces ending up in severe ADL limitations are: low education, poverty, preference for house care, and younger age of presentation for ADL limitations when compared to other ethnic groups, especially Caucasians. Since a higher frequency for household care is observed in this population. It would seem that the only real solution to this constant observation would be proper training between house members. Household members believe that it is their obligation to provide primary care to their elderly family members, as a sign a retribution for when they were taken care off during their childhood [28]. This phenomenon is observed in Hispanic families that have not been influenced by acculturation. Younger generations with higher levels of acculturation will be willing to seek proper help for their elderly household members in nursing homes or medical facilities, which in the end could prevent the severity of their ADL limitations.

Another social demographic factor that has been shown to be constant as a risk factor for ADL limitation is gender. Usually female Hispanic elderly have higher frequencies of ADL limitations [20, 36]. This is probably due to the high impact that religion, especially Catholicism, has on Hispanic society. In the Hispanic community about 68% are Catholic, 20% Protestants, 3% other Christian denominations, 1% other faiths, 8% secular and 8% don't participate in any religious community [37]; with these frequencies we can observe how Catholicism could have a great impact in their lifestyle. In fact, the Virgin Mary could be one of the mayor religious figures that could explain how Catholicism influences Hispanic older adults. The Virgin Mary is considered among several Latino women as an example on how life should be lived through saintliness [28].

The relationship between this self-sacrifice and the higher burden for ADL limitations is quite clear, especially in women. Gender differences have been observed between the elderly, where women are more likely to attend religious ceremonies when compared to men [37]. Although women have a higher attendance to religious ceremonies, women will usually not seek help even if they have ADL limitations in order to perform self-sacrifice so they could conserve their dignity and nobility [28]. This self-sacrifice among woman could also be influenced by low education. Those with low education will probably interpret their suffering with a positive explanation and will probably suffer in silence delaying proper medical help [37]. Not only do women have an image of self-sacrifice as a proper way of life; they have poor participation when making decisions. There seems to be no equal distribution when making decisions between genders in the Hispanic population, this term is called *machismo*. In Hispanic culture it is well seen that only men can make decisions in their family and it is their obligation to provide the necessary monetary income. This greatly impacts on how women could receive help from their disability since in the end it is their husband, for example, who will approve or not if she receives help in a nursing home. Nursing homes are usually seen as inappropriate in the Latino population. Elderly usually try to minimize their limitations to provide less burden and strain to the primary caregiver. It is known that the primary caregiver in the end will have disability at a younger age [35]. It is important to mention that not always will their primary caregiver be a younger household member. In many circumstances, their primary caregiver could in fact be their spouse. Interestingly, its wives that are usually more affected by their husband's disability than the other way around, once again the gender disparity is observed [38].

This gender disparity also reflects how women are more likely to be associated with more depressive symptoms than older men thus provoking further problems in their psychical health too. Probably women are more emotionally attached to their spouse´s health than vice versa, provoking them to have a greater risk for psychological distress. Men will usually seek help if their wife has certain functional limitation since they might not be prepared for the task of caregiving. Women will also seek help from their adult children and other relatives than from their husbands, provoking less stress for their husband. This less burden in their husband could help provoking less stress and prevent certain functional limitations [39]. It has been observed that only 26.2% of Mexican elderly have access to some king of medical insurance related to their work. Probably Latin American elderly face a higher obstacle since public health institutions have not considered a long term treatment or care for the elderly with ADL limitations [31].

This situation is not observed in those with higher income and access to a health insurance. Those with access to a health insurance will seek proper medical attention for their spouse's functional limitation and therefore will prevent developing depressive symptoms in the near future. By preventing psychological distress, psychical limitations can be prevented on the primary caregiver, in this case the spouse without functional limitations [39]. Although this seems like a great preventive measure, reality for this population is far worse, where informal jobs, no pension or access to proper medical care; social and cultural boundaries, and denial for proper medical help, may seem like there won't be any change creating an increased risk for functional limitations. This phenomenon will probably change in future generations which have higher levels of acculturation, where it has been observed that acculturation in Hispanic culture seems to be a protective factor. Probably because most will learn English, thus seeking better job opportunities and having access to better medical attention [66].

African-American Culture

African-American culture, like Hispanic culture, suffer from social economic difficulties with elevates the risk for disability. When compared with Whites, African American had a 5.78% higher incidence for disability (Figure 1, Dorothy D. Dunlop. 2005). This clearly demonstrates that this race may face risk factors not commonly presented in Caucasians that may lead to ADL limitations, functional limitations, and in the end, disability. Risk factors documented in this population are: age > 80, one or more physical limitations, and cardiovascular disease [30]. In fact, African-Americans have the highest percentage of ADL limitation, 24% versus 17% of the Caucasian population [30]. Some authors suggest that this risk begins before birth due to initial social locations which could provide certain opportunities and mark a pathway which could shape individuals' health, education, and career [40]. When one domain is related to produce disadvantage, this domain may produce disadvantages in subsequent domains. This can certainly be modified if the initial domain is prevented or intervened [41].

Probably the most consistent risk factor for functional decline is the lack of psychical activity [30, 34]. Certainly this can be explained when the population encounters low education and low income, having a higher risk for ADL disability and lack of psychical activity [36]. Although psychical inactivity is the highest risk factor for ADL limitation, it is not the only risk factor to be considered, since disability is considered to be caused by multiple factors. Other risk factors to be taken into account are the use of alternative medicine, which is quite frequent. Unlike the Asian population [42], alternative medicine could have a negative effect on the African-American population, resulting in higher risk for ADL limitations [43]. This attribution is probably the result of African-Americans, who prefer alternative medicine, including praying, from mainstream or modern medicine. Usually these patients seem to be sicker compared to the rest of the African-American population that do not use alternative medicine. Probably this greater level of comorbid conditions and complications is due to less preventive behaviors encountered in those who use alternative medicine; there is also less probability that this population will seek accurate medical help, in hope of receiving results with the use of alternative medicine [43].

African-Americans have less access to private medical insurance, which could also cause lack of proper medical attention and preventive measures. When compared to Caucasians, only 58% had employer-provided insurance coverage, which is quite a difference since 69% of Caucasians received employer-insurance [44]. Probably this racial disparity could be caused by the fact that African-Americans are less likely to have jobs that offer insurance by the employer. These job offers could be affected by social economic factors, like education and job discrimination, where African-Americans won't have the opportunity to seek jobs that offer insurance due to their education level. African Americans usually suffer from discrimination when seeking a job, 49% reported a lifetime occurrence of discrimination. This discrimination could lead to not being hired, being denied bank loans; 73% reported being treated with less courtesy or being called derogatory names at work [45]. This scenario clearly depicts the disparity African Americans face throughout life. This disparity is not always constant in this population. African-Americans with insurance from their job or spouse, excluding Medicare as their primary medical insurance, seemed to lower their risk for functional limitation. This way, resources were mobilized in a proper domain, having healthcare insurance, helping prevent subsequent domains that could in the end provoke lower levels of functional limitation [40].

Although social demographic factors have been mentioned to cause ADL limitations throughout this text, we must emphasize that modifiable risk factors have a higher burden in producing ADL limitations, especially in the African-American population. One of these modifiable risk factors that could affect the African-American population is being overweight or obese, this being measured by the body mass index. African-American women are more likely to be obese or overweight when compared to White women resulting in an increased risk for lower mobility limitation [46]. In fact, more than half of African-American women will be obese by the age of 40, [47]. Modifiable risk factors could also affect social demographic aspects. An example of this interaction could be seen with overweight African-American; being overweight appeared to weaken the benefit of additional years of education [46]. With less years of education, less are the opportunities for a better job and without a better job, those affected won't have access to a proper health insurance or won't have an adequate income incrementing their risk for disability. Even though, overweight and obesity are partially treated with psychical activity, it seems that this health promotion measure is not as protective as thought compared with White women [46]. This information implicates proper ethnic focused interventions to prevent or treat ADL limitations.

African Americans will usually seek help between their communities; this phenomenon seems to be constant among minorities, although this isn't always a rule. African Americans with higher education above the mean will usually have a negative interaction between family members and their community, in terms of seeking help for their disability [48]. As mentioned before, better education leads to better job opportunities and easier access to medical attention. Probably this population has better access and knowledge to preventive measures, leading to less ADL limitations.

Religion is also implicated in creating social support among the African American community. In fact, African Americans have the highest religious involvement according national surveys and polls. 89% of African Americans indicate that they are very involved or somewhat religious [37]. About 52% of African American are Baptist, 9% Methodist, 7% Pentecostal, 6% Catholic, 21% report other denominations and religions, and only 5% denied any religious affiliation [49]. An interesting observation is that only 20% of African Americans attend to Caucasian religious groups, which clearly demonstrates how religion is a synonym of community bonding between African-Americans [37]. African Americans see the act of praying as a form of alternative medicine, since indirectly by praying and attending religious ceremonies they will probably seek community help for certain conditions like ADL limitations. This observation between African-Americans is described in those with lower income and education. This population will probably spend more time investing in religious identities, especially those who are from southern states of the United States.

African Americans that assist church activities usually report church-based social support networks, such as direct aid and services which include help during illness, monetary loans, transportation, socio-emotional support, and group prayer; this clearly demonstrates why religion is so important in this community. Specifically ill older adults receive support by visitations from any member of the church, help with activities like chores, medical services, etc., this clearly concludes why disabled elderly with ADL limitations will probably dependent heavily on their religious community. Although a positive effect could be expected from this social network, not all is positive. In fact, religious managing of social and health problems will probably provoke negative health effects among the elderly. By having too much importance for religion as their primary support, older adults will probably end up with behaviors that inhibit seeking proper medical help and instead devote all their treatment exclusively by clergy or spiritual advisors [37, 50]. This could become detrimental for their well-being and health. Once again proper ethnic oriented interventions must be made in order to prevent or treat properly ADL limitations.

Asian and Pacific Islanders Culture

It has come to our observation that the world's highest life expectancy is found in Asia, especially in Hong Kong and Japan. Women from Hong Kong have a life expectancy of 82.5 years where women in Japan have a similar expectancy of 85.6 years [50]; this is probably influenced by the risk factors and environment they are exposed to throughout life. In fact, Asians in general seem to have less risk for disability, ADL limitations, or functional decline. Although this is true, the frequency may vary between Asian subpopulations. For example, Pacific Islanders have a higher incidence for ADL limitations when compared to Japanese or Asian Indians (Table 1). Probably this is due to specific risk factors that are encountered in each subpopulation, for example obesity which is higher in Pacific Islanders.

Psychical inactivity, depression, and comorbid conditions all play a role in the development of disability, although there is a strong risk factor to be considered to play a role in the natural history of disability, this is: diet. A clear example is the devotion to drink high doses of green team between the Asian populations, more precisely in Japan. Green tea consumption was found to lower the incidence of functional disability and was considered to be dose dependent [51]. In fact, in the Ohsaki Cohort 2006 study, Japanese diet compared to an animal pattern and high fat pattern diet resulted in a lower incidence of functional disability [52].

Although Japanese diet has been proven to be protective among this population, other factors should be included. Culture seems to have a constant impact on how the elderly reflect their perspective in ADL limitation. A clear example is the data analyzed through the U.S. Census Bureau in the 2006 American Community Survey. A result obtained through this analysis concluded that Asian and Pacific Islanders were less likely to receive help from institutions if they had ADL limitations compared to Non-Hispanic Whites [53]. Culture is the main explanation to this result; it was observed that those who spoke English were more likely to seek help from different institutions compared to Non-English Speakers. This phenomenon is similar to that described in the Hispanic population; it seems that language is a major barrier in the minorities that live in the United States of America; not to mention that those who were not citizens would not hesitate to seek medical attention [53]. Asian culture prefers to receive help from family members than to seek help in a nursing home [54]. It seems that Asian culture, like Hispanic culture, has excellent bonding between family members and would probably seek for help between family members if they had an ADL limitation. Family support is not always observed in Asian Americans when compared to Asian population migrating from their native country. Asian Americans will less likely seek help with their family members or among their social community. Asian Americans are more concerned about the negative impact they could provoke by seeking help leading to the perception of shame on oneself and worsening of the problem [48]. An important situation that has to be emphasized is the diverse subpopulations that exist in Asian culture; this includes Japanese, Vietnamese, Chinese, Hawaiian population, etc. It has been observed that some subpopulations have higher risk for disability compared to others. The subpopulations that have been observed to have a higher risk for disability are Hawaiian/ Pacific Islanders and Vietnamese [53]. The explanation to these findings are partially explained by the fact that Hawaiian/Pacific Islanders have a higher risk for obesity and type 2 diabetes, creating a risk for disability [55]. Vietnamese reflect a higher risk for disability, probably due to the fact that most Vietnamese elderly were exposed to the war during the 1960-70s and are now refugees in the United States [56]. Even though these two subpopulations have a higher risk for disability compared to other Asian cultures, in overall Asian subpopulations have less risk for disability compared to Caucasians [53], probably due to having a healthier lifestyle. We have mentioned diet as a protective factor, but what other protective factors are observed in this population? Besides a healthier lifestyle, Asians immigrants must meet certain minimum health standards imposed by the US government creating a positive selection effect [53].

When a healthier lifestyle is mentioned, we are not just taking into account the high green tea consumption that was mentioned earlier. Asians dietary habits include a low intake of saturated fat, red meat, and dairy, was well as a high intake of vegetables [53]. All these factors take a partial role in protecting this population for disability.

As a constant risk factor, socioeconomic status plays a major role in these subpopulations too. In fact, Japanese and Asian Indians were the subpopulations with the highest annual income. When Japanese were compared to Chinese in presenting disability, after adjustment of variables, the Japanese demonstrated a better disability outcome when compared to Chinese. This comparison is perhaps and effect influenced by the better socioeconomic status that is observed among the Japanese population [53].

Religion seems to influence in mortality and ADL limitations in the Asian population. During the analysis of the Chinese Longitudinal Healthy Longevity Surveys from 1998-2000, it was observed that 6% of religious participants had lower risk for mortality when compared to non-participants. This same relation was observed for ADL limitations, which were found to be less affected in religious participants. Some of the main factors that influenced Chinese to participate in religion were certain socioeconomic factors, such as an urban residency, unmarried, living alone, female gender, and age. Usually religious participants viewed their religious community as a bridge for social support; this could explain why some of the participants had lower risk for ADL limitations. It is also true that Chinese religion is largely influenced by alternative Chinese medicine, which could also have some positive effect on the elderly [42]. In conclusion, Asian who have a healthy lifestyle, with proper income, and social support may have less risk for ADL limitations, functional impairment, or disability. Contrary to Hispanics and African-Americans who seek social help, where these populations are negatively affected when seek social help instead of proper medical help.

Caucasian Culture

The proportion of elderly Caucasians in the United States is expected to decline from 87 percent in 1990 to 67 percent in 2050, probably this would be to an increase in the Hispanic and African-American elderly population and lower recent fertility [50].

Caucasians are less likely to suffer from ADL limitations compared to African-Americans or Hispanics. This had already been mentioned in previous sections in this chapter, after Asians; Whites seem to have less frequency for ADL limitations, functional decline, or disability. (Table 1) [57, 30]. Those that due suffer from ADL limitation are less likely to have worse scores when in a nursing home, compared to the Hispanic population [58]. White elderly with ADL limitations that evolve to disability with probably have a rapid increase in mortality when compared to African-American older adults [59]. Although this seems drastic, Whites will be less likely to present disability due to socioeconomic factors that could have a protective factor; one of these factors is health insurance. 79 percent of elderly Caucasians have private insurance, when only 39 percent of African-Americans and 36 percent of Hispanics had access to a private health insurance. Medicare is usually the sole source of medical insurance for these minorities, where only 13 percent of Whites used Medicare as their only source of health insurance [50]. This disparity could clearly explain why Whites seek help earlier for their ADL limitations, when compared to other races. The 1991-92 SIPP date clearly explains this idea, where those without private health insurance will be more likely to have disability than those covered by a private insurance, 49.6 percent of those not covered presented a severe functional limitation when compared to 29.5 percent of those with a private health insurance [60]. In fact, 9.3 percent of Caucasians referred their health status as excellent where only 5.5 percent of African-Americans referred the same status. On the contrast, 11 percent of Whites referred their health as being poor compared to 16.4 percent of African-Americans. Not only do Whites have a better perception of their health, but they are less likely to be affected by chronic conditions or even suffer less from their disability in the short course. Acute symptoms from disability, usually last 22.89 days for Whites when compared to 32.49 days in African-Americans [61]. This disparity could partially be explained by the income Whites have when compared to other races. White elderly make a median income of 15,276 dollars, where African-Americans make 8,031, and 9,253 for Hispanics 65 years or older [50]. This great gap influences the natural history of disability, where better access to health services and less dependence on family members could create less risk for future functional limitations leading to less disability in the White elderly.

Hispanics are more likely to be dependent on family members and will usually seek help when their family can no longer provide care; this is contrary to Caucasians who are usually independent and would seek help in an early stage. When compared to other races, only 17.1 percent of White elderly required assistance when compared to 25.2 percent for African-Americans and 25.3 percent for Hispanics [50], this clearly represents how Caucasians seem to be more independent. Although this could be beneficial in preventing further complications in functional limitations, complete lack of social connection has been known to increase the risk for all-cause mortality, heart disease mortality, and cancer mortality among Caucasians [62]. Cardiovascular disease and poverty seem to affect more often minorities than Caucasians resulting in a higher frequency of ADL limitation [30, 29]. Although it seems consistent that Whites have less risk for ADL limitations, this is partially true until a certain age. After age 75, there seems to be functional decline in Caucasian population, resulting in the end with higher instrumental ADL disability than black men and women [63]. Caucasians, like the rest of ethnicities, are also influenced by religious participation in society. White population who reported higher spirituality felt their health was in good conditions, although this population has greater education and income, which could affect their perception of good health [64].

Conclusion

Age may in the end be the highest and most important risk factor for disability [30], it is clear that race by itself plays a role as a risk factor for ADL limitations and/or disability. When race is influenced by comorbidities, environmental, and social factors, this theory seems to outstand even when compared to the theories explained in the introduction. Although age is the most important risk factor, there are racial differences that should be considered when referring to ADL limitations, functional impairment, or disability, especially African-Americans and Hispanics. The only real preventive measure should be encouraged during an early stage before becoming an older adult. Certain diet patterns, probably influenced by Asian culture, should be structured and implemented among young adults. Besides diet, physical activity may be a great preventive measure. Although we have an idea on which populations are likely more affected, this idea will quickly change because of the increase or decrease in certain races. Acculturation of future foreign populations will also have an effect on how certain races, like the Hispanic or Asian race will be affected by certain social risk factors for disability. Acculturation might change how different races seek help in the near future, as well as their religious and social participation among the community. Better opportunities and access to better education and jobs between different races could change the panorama that has been described.

References

[1] World Health Organization. Towards a common longuage for functioning, disability and health ICF Geneva: World Health Organization; 2002.

[2] Verbrugee L., Jet A. The disablement process. *Social Science and Medicine,* 1994; 38(1): p. 1-14.

[3] Gruenberg E. The Failure of Success. Milbank Memorial Fund Quarterly/*Health Society.* 1977; 55: p. 3-24.

[4] Fries J. Aging, natural death, and the compression morbidity. *The New England Journal of Medicine,* 1980; 303(3): p. 130-135.

[5] Fries J. The compression of morbidity: near or far? *Milbank Memorial Fund Quarterly*. 1989; 67: p. 208-232.

[6] Manton K. Changing concepts of morbidity and mortality in the elderly population. *The Milbank Memorial Fund Quarterly/ Health and Society,* 1982; 60(2): p. 183-244.

[7] Robine J., Michel J. "Looking forward to a general theory on population aging". *J. Gerontol. A. Biol. Sci. Med. Sci.,* 2004; 59(6): p. M590-M597.

[8] Gill T. M., Hardy S. E., Williams C. S. Underestimation of Disability in Community-Living Older Persons. *Journal American Geriatrics Society*, 2002; 50(9): p. 1492-1497.

[9] Min L. C., Elliott M. N., Wenger N. S., Saliba D. Higher Vulnerable Elders Survey Scores Predict Death and Functional Decline in Vulnerable Older People. *Journal American Geriatrics Society*, 2006; 54(3): p. 507-511.

[10] World Health Organization. World report on disability. [Online].; 2011 [cited 2014 10 15. Available from: http://whqlibdoc.who.int/publications/2011/9789240685215_eng.pdf?ua=1

[11] Bobak M., Kristenson M., Pikhart H., Marmot M. bmj.com. [Online].; 2004 [cited 2014 10 15. Available from: doi:10.1136/bmj.38202.667130.55.

[12] Arias-Merino E. D., Ortiz G. G., Flores-Saiffe M. E., Morales-Sanchez A., Maynard W., Velasquez-Brisuela I. E. Prevalence of cognitive impairment in Mexican elderly. In Alzhiemer's Disease: New Advances.; 2006. p. 667-671.

[13] Arias-Merino E., Mendoza-Ruvalcaba N., Ortiz G., Velázquez-Brizuela I., Meda-Lara R., Cueva-Contreras J. Physical function and associated factors in community-dwelling elderly people in Jalisco, Mexico. *Archives of Gerontology and Geriatrics*, 2012; 54(3): p. 271-278.

[14] Wolinsky F. D. STCCJJ. Consistency and change. *Journal of Aging and Health,* 1996; 8(155-182).

[15] Phelan E., Williams B., Pennix B., LoGerfo J., Leveille S. Activities of daily living function and disability in Older Adults in a randomized trial of the health enhancement program. *Journal of Gerontology Medical Sciences,* 2004; 59: p. 838-843.

[16] Schieman S., Plickert G. Functional limitations and changes in levels of depression among older adults: a multiple-hierarchy stratification perspective. *Journal of Gerontology Social Sciences,* 2007; 62: p. 36-42.

[17] Marengoni A., Von Strauss, Rizzuto D., Winblad B., Fratiglioni L. The impact of chronic multimorbidity and disability on functional decline and survival in elderly persons. A community-based longitudinal study. *Journal of Internal Medicine*, 2009; 265(2): p. 288-295.

[18] Thakral M., Shi L., Shmerling R., Bean J., Leveille S. A stiff Price top ay: does joint stiffness predict disability in an older population?. 2014;62(10): 1891-1899. *Journal of the American Geriatrics Society*, 2014; 62(10): p. 1891-1899.

[19] Griffith L., Raina P., Hongmei W., Stathokosta L. Population attributable risk for functional disability associated with chronic conditions in Canadian older adults. *Age and Ageing*, 2010; 39(6): p. 738-745.

[20] Snih S., Otternbacher J., Markides K., Kuo Y., Eschbach K., Goodwin J. The effect of obesuty on disability vs mortality in older americans. *Archives of Internal Medicine*, 2007; 167(8): p. 774-780.

[21] Tanimoto Y., Watanabe M., Sun W., Tanimoto K., Shishikura K., Sugiura y. Association of sarcopenia with functional decline un community-dwelling elderly subjects in Japan. *Geriatrics and Gerontology International,* 2013; 13(4): p. 958-963.

[22] Da Silva S., Scazufca M., Menezes P. Population impact of depression on functional disability in elderly: results from "Sao Paulo Ageing and Health Study" (SPAH). *European Archives of Psychiatry and Clinical Neuroscience,* 2013; 263(2): p. 153-158.

[23] Yamazaki S., Nakano K., Saito E., Yasumura S. Prediction of functional disability by depressive state among community-dwelling elderly in Japan: a prospective cohort study. *Geriatrics and Gerontology International,* 2012; 12(4): p. 680-687.

[24] Tomata Y., Watanabe T., Sugawara Y., Chou W., Kakizaki M., Tsuji I. Dietary patterns and incident functional disability in the elderly japanesse: The Ohsaki Cohort 2006 Study. *Journals of Gerontology Series A: Biological Sciences and Medical Sciences,* 2014; 69(7): p. 843-851.

[25] Mellqvist Fässberg M., Östling S., Braam A., Bäckman K., Copeland J., Ficher M. Functional disability and death wishes in older Europeans: results from the EURODEP concerted action. *Social Psychiatry and Psychiatric Epidemiology,* 2014; 49(9): p. 1475-1482.

[26] Reuben D. B., Leonard S. D. Office-based assessment of the older adult. [Online].; 2013 [cited 2014 10 15. Available from: http://www.uptodate.com/contents/office-based-assessment-of-the-older-adult.

[27] Tirodkal M. A., Song J., Chang R. W., Dunlop D. D., Chang H. J. Racial and Ethnic Differences in Activities of Daily Living Disability Among the Elderly: The Case of Spanish Speakers. *Arch. Phys. Med. Rehabil.,* 2008; 89(7): p. 1262-1266.

[28] Evans B. C., Belyea M. J., Coon D. W., Ume E. Activities of Daily Living in Mexican American Caregivers: The Key to Continuing Informal Care. *J. Fam. Nurs.,* 2012; 18(4): p. 439-466.

[29] Reyes-Ortíz C. A. The Disability-Poverty Connection in Older People. *Journal of the National Medical Association*, 91(2): p. 75-77.

[30] Shih V. C., Song J., Chang R. W., Dunlop D. D. Racial differences in activities of daily living limitation onset in older adults with arthritis: a national cohort study. *Arch. Phys. Med. Rehabil.,* 2005; 86: p. 1521-1526.

[31] Arias Merino E. D., Castillo Quezada M. D., Arias-Merino M. J. Funcionalidad física y discapacidad en el adulto mayor. In Arias-Merino E. D. Salud, Bienestar y Envejecimiento SABE Jalisco, Zona metropolitana de Guadalajara. Guadalajara: Editorial Universitaria; 2012. p. 727-731.

[32] Samper-Ternent R., Kuo Y. F., Ray L. A. Prevalence of Health Conditions and Predictors of Mortality in Oldest Old Mexican Americans and Non-Hispanic Whites. *J. Am. Med. Dir. Assoc.,* 2012; 13(3): p. 254–259.

[33] Wang Y., Wang Q. J. The prevalence of prehypertension and hypertension among US adults according to the new joint national committee guidelines: new challenges of the old problem. *Arch. Intern. Med.,* 2004; 164(19): p. 2126-2134.

[34] OECD. Pensions at a Glance 2013: OECD and G20 Indicators. [Online].; 2013. Available from: http://dx.doi.org/10.1787/pension_glance-2013-en.

[35] Hamman R. F., Mulgrew C. L., Baxter J., Shetterly S. M., Swenson C., Morgenstern N. E. Methods and Prevalence of ADL Limitations in Hispanic and Non-Hispanic White Subjects in Rural Colorado: The San Luis Valley Health and Aging Study. *Ann. Epidemiol.,* 1999; 9(4): p. 225–235.

[36] Dunlop D. D., Semanik P., Song J., Manheim L. M., Shih V., Chang R. W. Risk Factors for Functional Decline in Older Adults With Arthritis. *Arthritis and Rheumatism*, 2005; 52(4): p. 1274–1282.

[37] Chatters L. M., Nguyen A. W., Taylor R. J. Religion and Spirituality Among Older African Americans, Asians, and Hispanics. In Whitfield K., Baker T. Handbook of Minority Aging.: Spinger Publishing Company; 2013. p. 61-78.

[38] Ayotte B. J., Yang F. M., Jones R. N. Physical Health and Depression: A dyadic study of chronic health conditions and depressive

symptomatology in older couples. *Journal of Gerontology: Psychological Sciences Soc. Sci.,* 2010; 65(4): p. 438-448.

[39] Monserud M. A., Peek K. Functional Limitations and Depressive Symptoms: A Longitudinal Analysis of Older Mexican American Couples. *J. Gerontol. B. Psychol. Sci. Soc. Sc.,* 2014; 69(5): p. 743-762.

[40] Kail B. L., Taylor M. G. Cumulative Inequality and Racial Disparities in Health: Private Insurance Coverage and Black/ White Differences in Functional Limitations. *Journal of Gerontology B. Psychal. Sci. Soc. Sci.*, 2014; 69(5): p. 798-808.

[41] Ferraro K. F., Shippee T. P. Aging and Cumulative Inequality: How Does Inequality Get Under the Skin? *The Gerontologis*, 2009; 49(3): p. 333-343.

[42] Yi Z., Danan G., George L. Association of Religious Participation with Health and Survival Among the Oldest Old in China. [Online]. [cited 2014 10 14. Available from: http://paa2005.princeton.edu/papers/50633.

[43] Barner J. C., Bohman T. M., Brown C. M., Richards K. M. Use of Complementary and Alternative Medicine (CAM) for Treatment among African-Americans: A Multivariate Analysis. *Res. Social Adm. Pharm.,* 2010; 6(6): p. 169-208.

[44] Gould E., Hertel-Fernandez A. Early retiree and near-elderly health insurance in recession. *Journal of Aging and Social Policy*, 22: p. 172-187.

[45] Kessler R. C., Mickelson K. D., Williams D. R. The Prevalence, Distribution, and Mental Health Correlates of Perceived Discrimination in the United States. *Journal of Health and Social Behavior*, 1999; 40(3): p. 208-230.

[46] Latham K. Racial and Educational Disparities in Mobility Limitation Among Older Women: What is the Role of Modifiable Risk Factors? *Journal of Gerontology*, 2014; 69(5): p. 772-783.

[47] Wang Y., Beydoun M. A. The Obesity Epidemic in the United States-gender, age, socioeconomic, racial/ethnic, and geographic characteristics: A systemic review and meta-regression analysis. *Epidemiologic Reviews,* 29: p. 6-28.

[48] Lincoln K. D. Social Relationships and Health Among Minority Older Adults. In Whitfield K., Baker T. Handbook of Minority Aging.: Spinger Publishing Company, LLC; 2014. p. 42-44.

[49] Taylor R. J., Chatters L. M., Jackson J. S. Religious and Spiritual involvement among Older African Americans, Caribbean Blacks, and

non-Hispanic Whites: Findings from the National Survey of American Life. *Journal of Gerontology*, 2007; 62: p. 238-250.

[50] U.S. Bureau of the Census. 65+ in the United States.U.S. Current Population Reports, Special Studies, P23-190. Washington, DC:, Government Printing Office; 1996.

[51] Brenda W. J., Penninx H., Leveille S. Exploring the Effect of Depression on Physical Disability: Longitudinal Evidence From the Established Populations for Epidemiologic Studies of the Elderly. *Am. Journal of Public Health,* 1999; 89(9).

[52] Tomata, K., Kakizaki M., Nakaya N., Tsuboya T., Sone T., Kuriyama S., et al. Green tea consumption and the risk of incident functional disability in elderly Japanese: the Ohsaki Cohort 2006 Study. *The American Journal of Clinical Nutrition,* 2012; 95: p. 732–739.

[53] Fuller-Thomson E., Chi M. Older Asian Americans and Pacific Islanders with Activities of Daily Living (ADL) Limitations: Immigration and Other Factors Associated with Institutionalization. *Int. J. Environ. Res. Public Health*, 2012; 9: p. 3264-3279.

[54] Dong-soo S. Residential and caregiver preferences of older Korean Americans. *J. Gerontol. Nurs.*, 2008; 34(6): p. 48-54.

[55] Grandinetti A., Chan G. H. K., Chen R., Fujimoto W. Y., Rodriguez B. L., David Curb J. Prevalence of overweight and central adiposity is associated with percentage of indigenous ancestry among native Hawaiians. *International Journal of Obesity*, 1999; 23: p. 733-737.

[56] Mutchler J. E., Prakash A., Burr J. A. The Demography of Disability and the Effects of Immigrant History: Older Asians in the United States. *Demography,* 2007; 44(2): p. 251–263.

[57] Tirodkar M. A., Song J., Chang R. W., Dunlop D., Chang H. J. Racial and Ethnic Differences in Activities of Daily Living Disability Among the Elderly: The Case of Spanish Speakers. *Archives of Physical Medicine and Rehabilitation,* 2008; 89(7): p. 1262-1266.

[58] Mulrow C. D., Chiodo L. K., Gerety M. B., Lee S., Basu S., Nelson D. Function and medical comorbidity in south Texas nursing home residents Variations by ethnic group. *Journal Of The American Geriatrics Society*, 1996; 44(3): p. 279-284.

[59] Manton K. G., Stallard E. Health and Disability Differences Among Racial and Ethnic Groups. In Martin L. G., Soldo B. J. Racial and Ethnic Differences in the Health of Older Americans. Washington DC: National Academies Press; 1997. p. 43-105.

[60] U.S. Bureau of the Census. Americans with Disabilities: 1991-92, Current Population Reports, Household Economic Studies, P70-33. Washington, D.C: U.S. Government Printing Office, 1993.

[61] Escarce K. J. J., Puffer F. W. Black-White Differences in the Use of Medical Care by the Elderly: A Contemporary Analysis. In Martin L. G., Soldo B. J. Racial and Ethnic Differences in the Health of Older Americans.: National Academy Press; 1997. p. 183-209.

[62] Liu L., Newschaffer C. J. Impact of social connections on risk of heart disease, cancer, and all-cause mortality among elderly Americans: Findings from the Second Longitudinal Study of Aging (LSOA II). *Archives of Gerontology and Geriatr.,* 2011; 53(2): p. 168-173.

[63] Lin S. F., Beck A. N., Finch B. K. Black-White Disparity in Disability Among U.S. Older Adults: Age, Period, and Cohort Trends. *J. Gerontol. B. Psychol. Sci. Soc. Sci.*, 2014; 69(5): p. 784-797.

[64] Daaleman T. P., Perera S., Studenski S. A. Religion, Spirituality, and Health Status in Geriatric Outpatients. *Annals of Family Medicine,* 2004; 2(1): p. 49-53.

[65] De Souza L. R., Fuller-Thomson E. Acculturation and Disability Rates Among Filipino-Americans. *J. Immigrant Minority Health,* 2013; 15: p. 462–471.

[66] Sheffield K., Salinas J. English language use, health and mortality in older Mexican Americans. *J. Immigr. Minor. Health*, 2011 Apr.; 13(2) 232-238).

In: Activities of Daily Living (ADL)
Editor: Scott T. Lively

ISBN: 978-1-63463-913-2

Chapter 5

Evaluation of Hand Functionality during Activities of Daily Living (ADL): A Review

Margarita Vergara*[*], *Verónica Gracia-Ibáñez* and *Joaquín L. Sancho-Bru
Dpto. de Ingeniería Mecánica y Construcción.
Universitat Jaume I, Castelló, Spain

Abstract

Over a billion people (about 15% of the world's population) are estimated to be living with some disability, according to the World Health Organization (WHO). To protect the human rights of people with disability, a great effort is being made to unify the classification of disabilities. The WHO's International Classification of Functioning, Disability and Health (ICF) has become a recognized reference for classifying the degree of disability. Beyond the obvious limitations derived from the lack of body functions and structures, the ability to carry out Activities of Daily Living (ADL) is proposed in the ICF as the main

[*] Corresponding author: Margarita Vergara, Email: vergara@ uji.es, tel. +34 964728121, Fax +34 964728106, Departamento de Ingeniería Mecánica y Construcción, Avda. Sos Baynat, Universitat Jaume I, E12071 - Castelló, Spain

factor for classifying the degree of disability. According to the ICF, many of the deficiencies in the domains of activity and participation are focused on the upper limbs. Furthermore, hands are used for more than 5 hours a day only in ADL, excluding the time spent on working or sleeping. The functional evaluation of the hand in ADL is therefore essential to assess a person's degree of independence. Moreover, this evaluation is also important when it comes to examining the progress of rehabilitation programs or in clinical practice. At present, the functional evaluation of the hand is performed using qualitative methods like "Disabilities of the Arm, Shoulder and Hand" (DASH), some of which are highly subjective and valid only for a specific pathology. Objective methods like measuring passive ranges of angles or maximal forces for specific types of grasps are also used, but no objective measurements while performing ADL are considered. No consensus has been reached about a unified method to assess hand functionality while performing ADL, as might be desirable, so that professionals have to rely on their own experience to grade this.

The aim of this chapter is to review the role of the use of the hand in the ability to perform ADL, with special attention given to the evaluations of functionality that are being used to establish the degree of disability and to monitor the evolution in rehabilitation processes for different pathologies of the hand. Special attention is paid to analyzing the attempts that have been made to objectify the evaluation of hand disabilities through the analysis of grasp and handling, and their impact on current practice.

Keywords: functionality of the hand, activities of daily living, disability, rehabilitation

Abbreviations

ADL: Activities of Daily Living
AMA: American Medical Association
CRPD: Convention on the Rights of Persons with Disabilities
DASH: Disabilities of the Arm, Shoulder and Hand
ICF: International Classification of Functioning, Disability and Health
UN: the United Nations
WHO: World Health Organization.

1. Introduction

The human hand is one of the most complex and versatile mechanical systems. Its ability to grasp and manipulate is fundamental to be able to perform a great number of the activities of daily living (ADL) (Vergara, Sancho-Bru, Gracia-Ibáñez, & Pérez-González, 2014). Therefore, keeping the functionality of the whole hand is critical to ensure a full and autonomous life, not only in ADL but also in work life (Bullock, Zheng, Rosa, Guertler, & Dollar, 2013; Zheng, Rosa, & Dollar, 2011a). In fact, an impairment at the level of the metacarpophalangeal joints accounts for 54% of whole-person disabilities (Engelberg, 1988).

Because of the importance of the hand for performing ADL, the International Classification of Functioning, Disability and Health (ICF) of the World Health Organization (WHO) (WHO, 2001) established the ability to carry out ADL as the main factor for classifying the degree of disability. The WHO also emphasizes that the consequences of the disabilities depend to a large extent on the context: people with similar limitations, derived from the lack of body functions and structures, or with impairments that prevent them from performing ADL can experience a variety of difficulties in their lives, depending on their birthplace or place of residence.

Attempts have been made to universalize the protection of human rights for people with disability through the United Nations' (UN) Convention on the Rights of Persons with Disabilities (CRPD) (United Nations, 2006) and, more recently, through the World Report on Disability (WHO, 2011). However, this will be difficult to accomplish with the current procedures for establishing the degree of disability.

Nowadays, in the case of the hand, the functional assessment that is commonly used lacks objectivity. Focusing on the assessment of hand functionality, the tools used by the professionals are limited to goniometers for measuring passive ranges of motion (Ellis & Bruton, 2002; Engstrand, Krevers, & Kvist, 2011; Macionis, 2013; Norkin & White, 2009) and, in some cases, dynamometers for measuring maximal pinch and grip forces (R.W. Bohannon, 2001; Richard W. Bohannon, Peolsson, Massy-Westropp, Desrosiers, & Bear-Lehman, 2006; Mathiowetz, Weber, Volland, & Kashman, 1984; Rantanen, 1999; Roberts et al., 2011). With regard to the capabilities to perform ADL, subjective observations of such abilities are performed for a given list of ADL.

Furthermore, the assessment of the ability to perform ADL is useful not only to rate disability, but it is also of utmost importance to improve rehabilitation processes and surgical planning. Comprehending the implications of selecting a rehabilitative practice or a surgical procedure in the improvement of the functionality of the hand would make it possible to select the best option for the patient taking into account his or her habits and needs. Currently, professionals combine medical techniques like electromyography, radiography or tomography with subjective tests like the "Disabilities of the Arm, Shoulder and Hand" (DASH) test (De Smet, De Kesel, Degreef, & Debeer, 2007; Hudak, Amadio, & Bombardier, 2008). These are tools whose adequacy has not been demonstrated sufficiently in all cases (Changulani, Okonkwo, Keswani, & Kalairajah, 2008) and that have very low repeatability and a high level of subjectivity (Grao et al., 2006).

In this chapter a review of the role played by the hand in the ability to perform ADL is carried out. Special attention is paid to the evaluation of hand functionality in order to assess disability and to evaluate the progress achieved in rehabilitation processes or the restoration of hand functions after surgery.

2. ADL and Disabilities

Beyond the humanitarian aspect, worldwide disability figures can give an idea of the magnitude of the problem and its impact on the global economy. As reported by the UN, there are approximately 650 million persons with disabilities in the world (about 10% of the global population, the WHO reports over a million), with approximately 80% of them living in developing countries, under conditions of poverty and with restricted access to employment ("Mainstreaming disability in the development agenda," 2008). A report from the Australian Network on Disability (Deloitte Access Economics, 2011) estimated that "closing the gap between labor market participation rates and unemployment rates for people with and without disabilities by one-third would result in a cumulative $43 billion increase in Australia's gross domestic product over a decade in real dollar terms."[1]

Fortunately, the concept of disability, and the way people with disabilities are treated, has evolved a lot throughout history. The English Elizabethan Poor

[1] These estimates only account for the direct impact on gross domestic product, and do not include indirect effects from improved government fiscal balances and increased employment opportunities for careers.

Laws (1598-1601) expelled them from hospitals and monastery shelters for the poor. They were given a cap to collect alms, which is the origin of the term "handicap" and the reason why this term is considered offensive nowadays. During World War II they were considered genetically defective and were "mercy killed." In the 40s the perception changed: they were considered unfortunate and the objects of charity. In 1970s' different movements driven by the efforts of disabled people to acquire new rights and entitlements came into being. The problem started to be located not in the individual but in the environment (attitudes and barriers, lack of services). Since then, the social perspective, guided by international institutions like the UN or WHO, has improved as a result of the efforts made to try to get them to become independent, self-determined individuals and to recognize their equal rights and opportunities. The ICF (World Health Organization, 2002) substituted the concepts of "impairment," "disability" and "handicap" with those of "body functions and structures" and "activities-participation," highlighting the positive aspects (health) at the expense of the negative ones (weaknesses) and granting more importance to the socio-sanitary criteria to the detriment of those purely scientific ones (Hernandez-Milagro, Rodríguez-García, & Gerona-Galdame, 2008).

The meaning of having disabilities changes significantly depending on the person's place of birth. Developed countries, in general, have ratified and adhered to the CRPD. Policies in USA or Europe, although different, all guarantee minimum rights and promote integration. The specific actions carried out include training to promote societal integration, individual economic aids and social benefits, economic benefits to companies that favor the employment of people with disabilities, etc. And access to these aids depends on the degree of disability assessed by the relevant national agency. In countries that have ratified the CRPD and must therefore follow the precepts of the ICF, the criteria for assessing disability should be expected to be the same.

Nevertheless, due to the lack of objective tools, the desired uniformity does not seem to have been achieved. This leads to a different way of assessing disability in each country, so that estimates of the number of people with disabilities vary greatly depending on who publishes them. Many low-income African countries, for example, report prevalence rates under 5%, while high-income countries report rates on average in excess of 10%, some as high as 20% (Loeb, Eide, & Mont, 2008).

It is common to distinguish between assessment of work disability and assessment of disability. Work disability is a status of disease that prevents a person, either temporarily or permanently, from performing a professional activity. And disability, as defined by the WHO (World Health Organization, 2002), is a general term for the functional impairment resulting from injury or disease that limits the normal performance of ADL, also taking into account environment and participation restrictions.

Many countries, thus, usually have two different agencies to assess them, as well as different compensation programs for each case. The assessment of work disability, as expected, does not usually consider the ability to perform ADL, but only the ability to perform work activities. In the case of Spain, where the authors reside, such assessment consists in a quantitative evaluation using the American Medical Association (AMA) Guides as a reference. These Guides offer a system for rating impairment by introducing some data about body functions and structures, although they are not universally accepted and, in fact, are based largely on consensus rather than on scientific evidence (Holmes, 2013).

In order to rate the disability and determine the associated economic benefits, Spain relies fully on the percentage of whole-person impairment published in the AMA Guides, as do many other states. With regard to the assessment of disability, the ICF established the ability to carry out ADL as the main factor for classifying the degree of disability. However, the countries that adhered to the ICF are applying it to their regulations with huge differences in both time and procedure.

In the Spanish case, for example, the regulation that assesses disability came into force in 1999 and has still not been adapted to the ICF. Hence, the evaluation of disability does not take into account the limitations to perform ADL.

On the contrary, it uses the degree of impairment of body structure, which is directly linked with a functional deficiency through the AMA Guides. In addition, in 2006, a new law came into force to introduce the concept of dependency: the functional inability to carry out ADL and thus requiring the care of a third person. This assessment is the first attempt made in Spain to consider the ability to perform ADL through the ICF of the WHO, and also provides for economic benefits, which complement the benefits stemming from the recognition of disability of the previous law.

3. ADL in Rehabilitation or Clinical Evaluation

Assessing the ability to perform ADL is also important to be able to establish the level of improvement in rehabilitation processes and to choose the best clinical treatments for enhancing the capability to perform ADL and therefore gain autonomy and happiness. The rehabilitation might also be achieved in a shorter time, with substantial cost savings.

Many studies have examined the evolution of the ability to perform ADL in patients under clinical or rehabilitation treatments (Bartolo et al., 2012; K. Bendstrup, Ingemann Jensen, Holm, & Bengtsson, 1997; Chemerinski, Robinson, & Kosier, 2001). Movement skills such as grasp and manipulation seem to be directly related with the capability to perform ADL.

However, the capacity to perform ADL depends not only on physical capacities, but also on the performance of the cognitive function as well as on the person's participation or social skills. Knowledge of these relationships is of great importance in rehabilitation practice in order to guide interventions towards meaningful targets (Coster, Haley, Jette, Tao, & Siebens, 2007). In fact, rehabilitation processes seem to be more effective when ADL are trained directly, for example with the support of virtual reality technology (Guidali et al., 2011; Lee et al., 2003). Therefore, assessing the ability to perform ADL is a widely-used method in quantifying both physical and psychological damage. The paradigm of using this method is probably in cases of strokes and geriatric rehabilitation.

For example, in strokes, the ability to perform ADL has long been considered a measure to assess their progress (Chiou & Burnett, 1985; Hellström, Lindmark, Wahlberg, & Fugl-Meyer, 2003) and the rehabilitation exercises that are used are designed to improve ADL (Mehrholz, Kugler, & Pohl, 2011). In the case of geriatric rehabilitation, different scales are used to verify the improvements in the ability to perform the ADL (Demers, Desrosiers, Nikolova, Robichaud, & Bravo, 2010).

Furthermore, the assessment of the ability to perform ADL is used not only in general assessments but also to study specific pathologies or diseases. As an example, it has been used in assessing loss of vision in the elderly (Kempen, Ballemans, Ranchor, Van Rens, & Zijlstra, 2012), in assessing the improvements afforded by rehabilitation in older people with femoral neck fractures (Stenvall, Olofsson, Nyberg, Lundström, & Gustafson, 2007) or in other conditions such as chronic obstructive pulmonary disease (K.E.

Bendstrup, Ingemann Jensen, Holm, & Bengtsson, 1997). Similarly, assessing the ability to perform ADL is not only used to evaluate the improvement in cases of physical illness, but is also widely used in cases of neurological disorders such as dementia (Littbrand, Stenvall, & Rosendahl, 2011; Liu et al., 2007; Mioshi, Hodges, & Hornberger, 2013) or Alzheimer (Ávila et al., 2004; G.A. Marshall et al., 2011).

In most studies the way of measuring the ability to perform ADL is often subjective, according to different scales (Chiou & Burnett, 1985; Hellström et al., 2003; Stenvall et al., 2007). However, there are some cases where attempts have been made to use objective means of measuring the kinematic ability to carry out ADL. Henmi et al. (2006) used an optical three-dimensional motion analysis system when monitoring the kinematics of the neck and upper limbs while performing ADL.

Hemmerich et al. (2006) measured the kinematics of the hip, knee and foot while performing ADL using a 6 degree-of-freedom electromagnetic tracking system. Similarly, Samuel et al. (Urwin, Kader, Caplan, St Clair Gibson, & Stewart, 2013) used an electrogoniometer to evaluate the kinematics of the knee while performing ADL. Electrogoniometry has also been used to study the effect of rigid cervical collar height on the full, active and functional range of motion during fifteen ADL (Miller, Bible, Jegede, Whang, & Grauer, 2010).

4. The Role of the Hand in the Ability to Perform ADL

The analysis of specific grasps is a common practice in the biomechanical and rehabilitation fields (Connell, McMahon, Watkins, & Eng, 2014; Pérez-González et al., 2012; Podobnik, Mihelj, & Munih, 2009; Sancho-Bru, Pérez-González, Vergara, & Giurintano, 2003). The selection of these grasps as being representative of hand behaviour is performed in many cases with a lack of scientific rigor (Kilbreath & Heard, 2005; Zheng, Rosa, & Dollar, 2011b; Sollerman & Ejeskar, 1995). In a previous study (Vergara et al., 2014), the authors performed a field study (on a representative sample of the adult population of a developed country) aimed at providing knowledge on the frequency and duration of use of the different types of grasp when performing different ADL. These data can be very useful in the assessment of the functional recovery of the hand during rehabilitation after injury or disease, for making clinical decisions and for prostheses design (Sollerman & Ejeskar, 1995), among others. The ADL were classified into 8 areas (food preparation, feeding, personal care, housekeeping, shopping, driving and transport, leisure, and others that are difficult to classify like talking on the phone, moving around the house, etc.), in an attempt to represent the most common ADL carried out by adult people. These areas represent a total of 8.42 hours on average per day (according to the data reported by the American Time Use Survey) and more than 5 hours using hands (Vergara et al., 2014). Work time was not considered.

The results drawn from this study showed that the areas in which hands are used for more time are feeding and leisure and the most frequently used grasp, overall, is the pinch. However, though almost all grasps are used in all areas, they are used with different frequencies or durations; for example, the pinch is used to a great extent in areas like food preparation or leisure, but less in driving.

It is remarkable that the most widely used grasps involve the thumb in opposition to the palmar side of the fingers (thumb in abduction), whereas the least used grasps either do not involve the thumb at all or the thumb is in opposition to the lateral side of the fingers. It is also significant that the amount of time in which both hands are used simultaneously is greater than when they are used alone, regardless of whether it is the right or the left hand. Grasps requiring more dexterity, like the pinch, are widely used by the right hand in the right-handed population, while other helping grasps, like non-prehensile grasp, are often used by the left hand to help the right hand.

In order to make these data more useful for disability assessment, it is very convenient to identify the activities of the ICF established by the WHO in which the hand is involved and which grasps are more frequently used in those activities. We have analyzed the activities of Part 1 "Functioning and Disability" of the ICF (Part 2 "Contextual Factor" refers to "Environmental and Personal Factors"). Part 1 is divided into two components: a) Body Functions and Structures, and b) Activities and Participation. Body functions are the physiological functions of body systems (including psychological functions), whereas Body structures are anatomical parts of the body such as organs, limbs and their components. In order to consider the role of the hand in the ability to perform ADL, only the second component, i.e., Activities and Participation, has been analyzed.

Table 1 shows all the chapter headings for this component as well as the subdivisions (items) until the level of three-digit codes, according to the ICF classification.

Table 1. Level of involvement of the hand in "Activities and Participation" of the ICF

	LEVEL		
ACTIVITIES AND PARTICIPATION	A	B	C
Chapter 1 Learning and applying knowledge			
Purposeful sensory experiences			
d110 Watching			■
d115 Listening			■
d120 Other purposeful sensing		■	
d129 Purposeful sensory experiences, other specified and unspecified		■	
Basic learning			
d130 Copying		■	
d135 Rehearsing		■	
d140 Learning to read		■	
d145 Learning to write		■	
d150 Learning to calculate		■	
d155 Acquiring skills		■	
d159 Basic learning, other specified and unspecified		■	
Applying knowledge			
d160 Focusing attention			■
d163 Thinking			■
d166 Reading		■	
d170 Writing		■	
d172 Calculating		■	
d175 Solving problems			■
d177 Making decisions			■
d179 Applying knowledge, other specified and unspecified			■
d198 Learning and applying knowledge, other specified			■
d199 Learning and applying knowledge, unspecified			■
Chapter 2 General tasks and demands			
d210 Undertaking a single task		■	
d220 Undertaking multiple tasks		■	
d230 Carrying out daily routine		■	
d240 Handling stress and other psychological demands			■
d298 General tasks and demands, other specified		■	
d299 General tasks and demands, unspecified		■	
Chapter 3 Communication			
Communicating - receiving			
d310 Communicating with - receiving - spoken messages			■
d315 Communicating with - receiving - nonverbal messages			■
d320 Comm. with - receiving - formal sign language messages			■
d325 Communicating with - receiving - written messages		■	

	LEVEL		
ACTIVITIES AND PARTICIPATION	A	B	C
d329 Communicating - receiving, other specified and unspecified			
Communicating - producing			
d330 Speaking			
d335 Producing nonverbal messages			
d340 Producing messages in formal sign language			
d345 Writing messages			
d349 Communication - producing, other specified and unspecified			
Chapter 3 Communication(cont.)			
Conversation and use of communication devices and techniques			
d350 Conversation			
d355 Discussion			
d360 Using communication devices and techniques			
d369 Conversation and use of comm. devices and tech., other specified and unspecified			
d398 Communication, other specified			
d399 Communication, unspecified			
Chapter 4 Mobility			
Changing and maintaining body position			
d410 Changing basic body position			
d415 Maintaining a body position			
d420 Transferring oneself			
d429 Changing and maintaining body position, other specified and unspecified			
Carrying, moving and handling objects			
d430 Lifting and carrying objects			
d435 Moving objects with lower extremities			
d440 Fine hand use			
d445 Hand and arm use			
d449 Carrying, moving and handling objects, other specified and unspecified			
Walking and moving			
d450 Walking			
d455 Moving around			
d460 Moving around in different locations			
d465 Moving around using equipment			
d469 Walking and moving, other specified and unspecified			
Moving around using transportation			
d470 Using transportation			

Table 1. (Continued)

	LEVEL		
ACTIVITIES AND PARTICIPATION	A	B	C
d475 Driving	■		
d480 Riding animals for transportation	■		
d489 Moving around using transportation, other specified and unspecified		■	
d498 Mobility, other specified		■	
d499 Mobility, unspecified		■	
Chapter 5 Self-care			
d510 Washing oneself	■		
d520 Caring for body parts	■		
d530 Toileting	■		
d540 Dressing	■		
d550 Eating	■		
d560 Drinking	■		
d570 Looking after one's health		■	
d598 Self-care, other specified	■		
d599 Self-care, unspecified	■		
Chapter 6 Domestic life			
Acquisition of necessities			
d610 Acquiring a place to live		■	
d620 Acquisition of goods and services		■	
d629 Acquisition of necessities, other specified and unspecified		■	
Chapter 6 Domestic life (cont.)			
Household tasks			
d630 Preparing meals	■		
d640 Doing housework	■		
d649 Household tasks, other specified and unspecified	■		
Caring for household objects and assisting others			
d650 Caring for household objects	■		
d660 Assisting others	■		
d669 Caring for household objects and assisting others, other specified and unspecified	■		
d698 Domestic life, other specified		■	
d699 Domestic life, unspecified		■	
Chapter 7 Interpersonal interactions and relationships			
General interpersonal interactions			
d710 Basic interpersonal interactions			■
d770 Intimate relationships (include sexual relationships)		■	

	LEVEL		
ACTIVITIES AND PARTICIPATION	A	B	C
d729 General interp. interactions, other specified and unspecified			
Particular interpersonal relationships			
d730 Relating with strangers			
d740 Formal relationships			
d750 Informal social relationships			
d760 Family relationships			
d770 Intimate relationships			
d779 Particular interpersonal relationships, other specified and unspecified			
d798 Interp. interactions and relationships, other specified			
d799 Interpersonal interactions and relationships, unspecified			
Chapter 8 Major life areas			
Education			
d810 Informal education			
d815 Preschool education			
d820 School education			
d825 Vocational training			
d830 Higher education			
d839 Education, other specified and unspecified			
Work and employment			
d840 Apprenticeship (work preparation)			
d845 Acquiring, keeping and terminating a job			
d850 Remunerative employment			
d855 Non-remunerative employment			
d859 Work and employment, other specified and unspecified			
Economic life			
d860 Basic economic transactions			
d865 Complex economic transactions			
d870 Economic self-sufficiency			
d879 Economic life, other specified and unspecified			
d898 Major life areas, other specified			
d899 Major life areas, unspecified			
Chapter 9 Community, social and civic life			
d910 Community life			
d920 Recreation and leisure			
d930 Religion and spirituality			
d940 Human rights			
d950 Political life and citizenship			
d998 Community, social and civic life, other specified			
d999 Community, social and civic life, unspecified			

The following gradation was considered: "A" means that there is a direct and unpreventable involvement of the hand; "B" means that it is indirectly involved, and "C" means no involvement at all. As an example, "A" is selected for activities such as "Dressing" (d540) or "Eating" (d550), as hands are essential in these activities; "B" is used for "Learning to read" (d140), which involves hands indirectly to hold a book or pass the pages; and "C" is considered for Interpersonal relationships, as it is assumed that interacting socially does not necessarily involve contact or actions with the hands.

5. The Present Status of the Assessment of Functionality of the Hand

Regardless of whether the evaluation of the functionality of the hand is required to assess disability or to assess rehabilitation processes and clinical treatments, the first step is always to identify the pathology or disease that causes the loss of functionality, which may be injuries specific to the hand or other diseases that can affect functionality indirectly. This is usually performed by medical professionals using clinical diagnostic tests (X-rays, Computed Tomography, Electromyography, etc.). This diagnosis should be carried out in accordance with the WHO's International Classification of Disabilities (WHO, 2010), and allows the medical team to gain an idea of what kind of actions might be hindered by the pathology, which can be helpful in order to assess the level of functionality of the hand. However, at this point the need for tools and methodologies capable of taking into account the subject's particularities arises. These tools should ideally be valid for any disease or pathology affecting the hands, and should be able to assess the subject's loss of hand functionality both objectively and accurately.

As regards the assessment of disability, the WHO's ICF (WHO, 2001) requires taking into account both the "Functioning and Disability" and the "Contextual Factors." As said before, the first component includes both the "Body Functions and Structures," i.e., structural and functional impairment, and "Activities and Participation," i.e., the ability to perform ADL. The methods currently used to assess the "Body Functions and Structures" for the case of the hand are limited to measuring passive ranges of motion with goniometry (Ellis & Bruton, 2002; Engstrand et al., 2011; Macionis, 2013; Norkin & White, 2009) or maximal forces in cylindrical and pinch grasps with dynamometers (R.W. Bohannon, 2001; Richard W. Bohannon et al., 2006;

Mathiowetz et al., 1984; Rantanen, 1999; Roberts et al., 2011). The "Activity and Participation" assessment is limited to the observation of specific actions that are intended to be representative of ADL, and questionnaires administered to the patients regarding their skills when performing ADL (Jefatura del Estado España, 2006; S.C. Marshall et al., 2007). The assessment of hand functionality during rehabilitation processes or clinical planning is usually performed through highly subjective specific tests or scales for each pathology (Amirjani, Ashworth, Olson, Morhart, & Chan, 2011; Backman & Mackie, 1995; Brogardh, Persson, & Sjolund, 2007), combined with the objective measurement of passive ranges of motion using goniometers, and maximal cylindrical or pinch grasping forces using dynamometers. With regard to the use of goniometry, institutions that have to assess disability have a latent problem because measurements are highly dependent on the operator's intention. In the measurement of the passive range of motion, an orthopaedic surgeon can force a joint more than a physical therapist or an assessment professional because of their professional experience and depending on what he expects to obtain (de Carvalho, Mazzer, & Barbieri, 2012). There is an interest to link objective measurements of "normality" with the ability to perform ADL (Faria-Fortini, Michaelsen, Cassiano, & Teixeira-Salmela, 2011; Hume, Gellman, McKellop, & Brumfield, 1990). Functional evaluators welcome any objective tool allowing them to do so, even when it is very simple (Soler & Rizos, 2006). This is the case of a protocol that is widely used in Spain that consists in using a dynamometer to record the maximum force of the cylinder grasp and distal and lateral pinch and to estimate fatigue from a series of forces and times. It is also common practice to compare ranges of motion and maximal grasping forces of the healthy and affected hands of a subject or with respect to values taken from normality databases (Cano-de la Cuerda, Águila-Maturana, & Macías-Jiménez, 2008; Lorenzo-Agudo, Santos-García, & Sánchez-Belizón, 2007).

Some previous studies have reviewed the tests and scales used in clinical or rehabilitation practice (Metcalf, Adams, Burridge, Yule, & Chappell, 2007; Lemmens, Timmermans, Janssen-Potten, Smeets, & Seelen, 2012; Lin, Chuang, Wu, Hsieh, & Chang, 2010). Metcalf et al. (2007) identified twenty-five different methods for conducting the clinical assessment of the upper limbs within the framework of the WHO's ICF. Thus, there are many tests available and medical professionals have to choose the most suitable for evaluating a specific pathology or illness, based on studies conducted to evaluate the sensitivity and validity for that specific pathology.

Table 2. Review of assessments used for the functionality of the upper limb

Name of the assessment	Description	For specific diseases	Valid/Specific for hand
Action Research Arm Test	Assesses upper limb functioning using observation. It is a 19-item measure (grasps and gross arm movement).	✓	✓
Arthritis Hand Function Test	Assesses hand strength and dexterity in patients with arthritis.	✓	✓
Box and Block Test	Assesses unilateral gross manual dexterity in cases of Stroke, Multiple sclerosis, Neuromuscular disorders, etc.	✓	✓
Conchin Hand Function Scale	Assesses functional ability of the hand in patients with arthritis, sclerosis, etc. 18-item questionnaire.	✓	✓
DASH	Assesses the loss of functionality in patients with upper limb disorders. 30-item questionnaire about ADL.	✓	✓
Frenchay Activities Index	Assesses a broad range of activities of daily living in patients recovering from stroke.	✓	
Fugl-Meyer Test	Assesses motor recovery after stroke. 226 items across 5 domains.	✓	✓
Jebsen Test	Assesses a broad range of uni-manual hand functions required in ADL. 7-10 items timed.		✓
Michigan Hand Questionnaire	Assesses patient's perception of hand function, pain and satisfaction on ADL. 37 items.		✓
Nine Hole Peg Text	Measures finger dexterity by taking pegs and placing them into holes following the instructions.	✓	✓
Purdue Pegboard Test	Assesses the dexterity of the hand, gross movements and fine "fingerprint" dexterity, in patients with Parkinson's disease.	✓	✓
Quality of Upper Extremity Skills Test	Assesses movement patterns and hand function in children with cerebral palsy from ages 18 months to 8 years.	✓	✓
Sollerman Test	Assesses hand function while performing ADL in Spinal Cord Injury patients. Scores timed range from 0-80.	✓	✓
Strength-Dexterity Test	Assesses the dynamic pinch performance used in ADL by testing strength and dexterity in some actions.		✓
Worf Motor Function Test	Assesses upper extremity motor ability through timed and functional tasks. It consists of 17-21 items.	✓	✓

	ICF domain:				Type of data		
Name of the assessment	Body Functions and Structures	Activities and Participation	ADL capabilities directly inferred from the outcomes	Use of instrumentation	Objective data	Observation	Studies of reliability
Action Research Arm Test	✓*	✓	✓	✓		✓	✓
Arthritis Hand Function Test	✓	✓*		✓"	✓		✓
Box and Block Test	✓*	✓		✓	✓		✓
Conchin Hand Function Scale		✓	✓			✓	✓
DASH		✓	✓			✓	✓
Frenchay Activities Index		✓	✓			✓	✓
Fugl-Meyer Test	✓					✓	✓
Jebsen Test		✓	✓	✓"	✓	✓	✓
Michigan Hand Questionnaire		✓	✓			✓	✓
Nine Hole Peg Text	✓			✓	✓		✓
Purdue Pegboard Test	✓			✓	✓		✓
Quality of Upper Extremity Skills Test	✓					✓	✓
Sollerman Test		✓	✓	✓"	✓	✓	✓
Strength-Dexterity Test	✓	✓	✓	✓	✓		✓
Worf Motor Function Test	✓*	✓	✓	✓"		✓	✓

✓"means that instrumentation is required, but common things can be used and it is free.
✓* means that the level of assessing this domain is relative.

For example, Lin et al. (2010) analysed the responsiveness and validity of three dexterous function measurements in stroke rehabilitation. Lemmens et al. (2012) systematically reviewed the instruments used for assessing arm-hand skilled performance in patients with stroke or cerebral palsy. The instruments identified were mainly tests and scales, only applicable in most cases to stroke or cerebral palsy. Although many instruments exist to assess capacity and perceived performance, a lack of instruments for assessing actual performance was reported. Lemmens also evidenced a dearth of instruments intended to be applied simultaneously in both components of the ICF, "Body Functions and Structures" and "Activities and Participation."

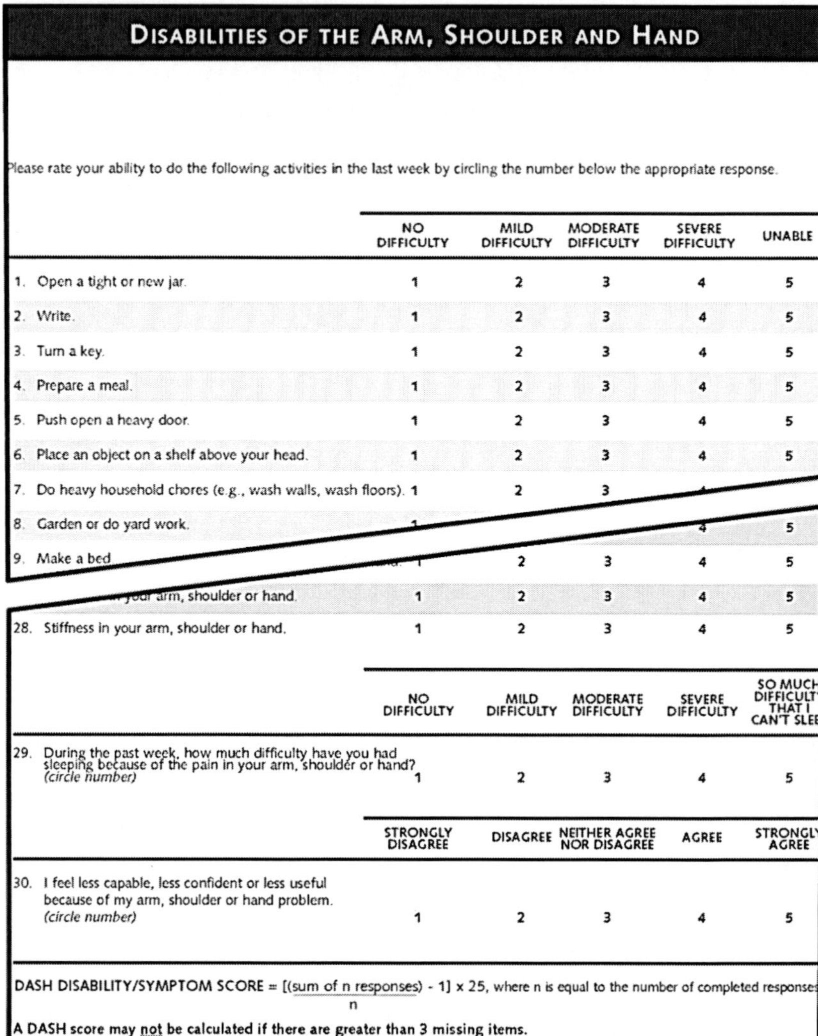

DISABILITIES OF THE ARM, SHOULDER AND HAND

Please rate your ability to do the following activities in the last week by circling the number below the appropriate response.

	NO DIFFICULTY	MILD DIFFICULTY	MODERATE DIFFICULTY	SEVERE DIFFICULTY	UNABLE
1. Open a tight or new jar.	1	2	3	4	5
2. Write.	1	2	3	4	5
3. Turn a key.	1	2	3	4	5
4. Prepare a meal.	1	2	3	4	5
5. Push open a heavy door.	1	2	3	4	5
6. Place an object on a shelf above your head.	1	2	3	4	5
7. Do heavy household chores (e.g., wash walls, wash floors).	1	2	3		
8. Garden or do yard work.				4	5
9. Make a bed		2	3	4	5
...your arm, shoulder or hand.	1	2	3	4	5
28. Stiffness in your arm, shoulder or hand.	1	2	3	4	5

	NO DIFFICULTY	MILD DIFFICULTY	MODERATE DIFFICULTY	SEVERE DIFFICULTY	SO MUCH DIFFICULTY THAT I CAN'T SLEEP
29. During the past week, how much difficulty have you had sleeping because of the pain in your arm, shoulder or hand? *(circle number)*	1	2	3	4	5

	STRONGLY DISAGREE	DISAGREE	NEITHER AGREE NOR DISAGREE	AGREE	STRONGLY AGREE
30. I feel less capable, less confident or less useful because of my arm, shoulder or hand problem. *(circle number)*	1	2	3	4	5

DASH DISABILITY/SYMPTOM SCORE = [(sum of n responses) - 1] x 25, where n is equal to the number of completed responses
n

A DASH score may not be calculated if there are greater than 3 missing items.

Figure 1. Items of the DASH Questionnaire. Figure extracted from the Institute for Work & Health website (http://dash.iwh.on.ca/home). The questionnaire was developed by them, jointly with the American Academy of Orthopedic Surgeons (AAOS).

Table 2 shows a description of 15 of the several tests and scales used in clinical and rehabilitation assessment. Actual assessments range from questionnaires with no objective data measured, such as the DASH (Figure 1) or Quality of Upper Extremity Skills tests, to questionnaires where body functions are tested using data that are objective but were not obtained during the performance of ADL, such as the Purdue Pegboard or Nine Hole Peg tests (Figure 2).

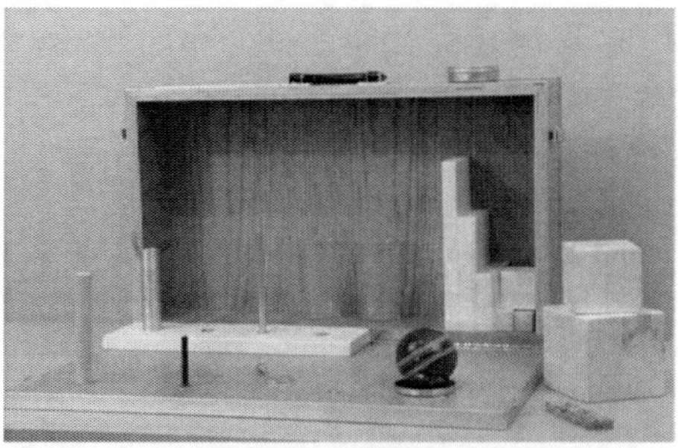

Action Research Arm Test

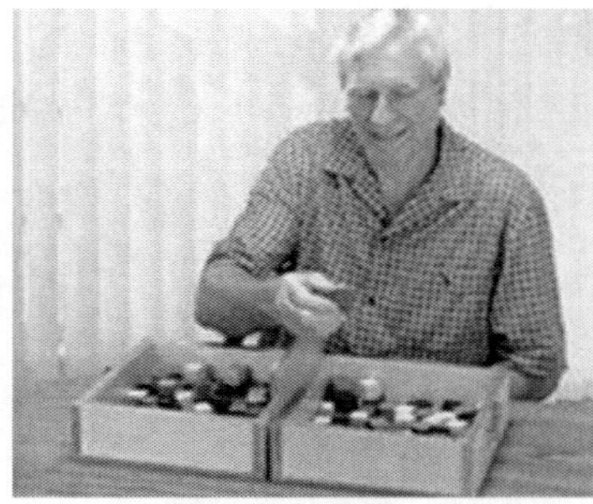

Box and Block Test

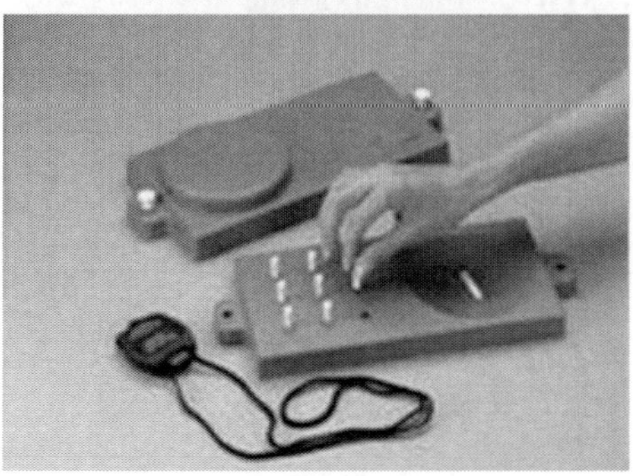

Nine Hole Peg Test

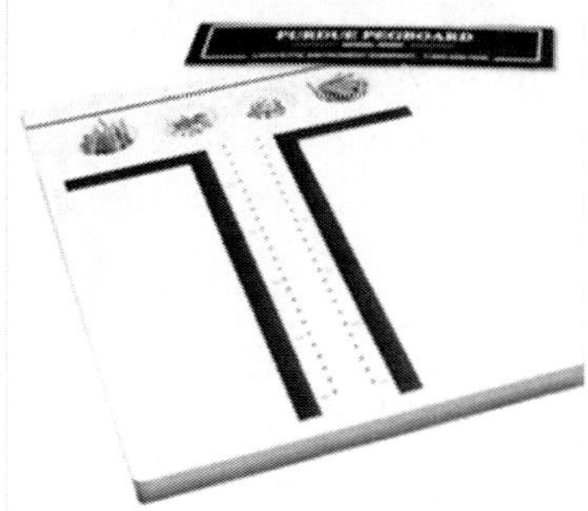

Purdue Pegboard Test

Figure 2. Images of instrumentation used in different assessment scales or tests.

Only some of the tests presented evaluate the ability to perform ADL through observation, such as the Sollerman or Jebsen tests. Furthermore, there are very few experimental studies dealing with the objective assessment of the intact upper limb function while performing ADL (Aizawa et al., 2010; Alt Murphy, Sunnerhagen, Johnels, & Willén, 2006; Butler et al., 2010; Chen, Xiong, Huang, Sun, & Xiong, 2010; Magermans, Chadwick, Veeger, & van der Helm, 2005; Sheikhzadeh, Yoon, Pinto, & Kwon, 2008; van Andel, Wolterbeek, Doorenbosch, Veeger, & Harlaar, 2008), and even fewer that refer specifically to the hand (Luker, Aguinaldo, Kenney, Cahill-Rowley, & Ladd, 2014; Oess, Wanek, & Curt, 2012; Rahman, Fai, & Ming, 2013). And there are also few studies assessing the pathological upper limb (Molina Rueda et al., 2012; Murgia, Kyberd, & Barnhill, 2010) or hand (Wade, Chen, &

Winstein, 2014) functionality while performing ADL. Moreover, these studies are biased to a particular disease or to a specific activity. For example, Murgia et al. (2010) studied the use of a kinematic indicator to assess the upper extremity status of distal radius fracture patients, but they only considered the activity of page-turning. And Molina et al. (2012) registered the kinematics and electromyography of the upper limb of patients with upper extremity hemiparesis due to stroke, during the activity of drinking from a glass.

Conclusion

The objective assessment of hand functionality while performing ADL, from experimental data registered in healthy and pathological hands, is a field that still requires a great deal of work. Given the importance of assessing the functionality of the hand, both in the field of disability evaluation and in rehabilitation and clinical practice, and taking into account the analysis of the present status, two matters become obvious:

Firstly, the analysis of hand functionality is very important in the context of the performance of ADL, particularly within the framework of the WHO's ICF. As more countries ratify the UN Convention, there is an increasing interest to improve disability assessment in order to follow the precepts of the WHO. Recent literature also reveals a growing interest to evaluate the patient's progression during rehabilitation processes for specific diseases based on the evolution of the ability to perform ADL. The development of a tool to assess the functionality of the hand during the different ADL required for the patient's autonomy and valid for any disease would be highly desirable.

Secondly, actual procedures to assess hand functionality while performing ADL present a lack of objectivity that makes it difficult to infer the patient's progress in the ability to carry out ADL. Moreover, the tests or scales available today are only applicable for specific diseases. The conclusion is that there is a need for a general and objective tool to assess the functionality of the hand.

New tools for functional assessment are called for, and especially scales than can be applied simultaneously in both components of the ICF: "Body Functions and Structures" and "Activities and Participation." Such a tool could link the two components (the lack of functionality in performing ADL due to the occurrence of a structural impairment) and would simplify the assessments, thus making them more realistic (the maximum range of motion is not always required to perform ADL).

Finally, although the ability to grasp and handle is essential to be able to perform ADL, not many attempts have been made to objectify the evaluation of hand disabilities through the analysis of grasp and handling. It is true that there are some studies in the field of rehabilitation that use grasp capabilities to improve the ability to perform ADL, mainly in stroke patients. However, the use of grasps in ADL has seldom been linked as a way to measure and assess the functionality of the hand.

Acknowledgments

We thank the Universitat Jaume I for funding through the projects P1·1B2013-33 and P1·1B2014-10, in which this research is partially included.

References

Aizawa, J., Masuda, T., Koyama, T., Nakamaru, K., Isozaki, K., Okawa, A., & Morita, S. (2010). Three-dimensional motion of the upper extremity joints during various activities of daily living. *Journal of Biomechanics*, *43*(15), 2915–22.

Alt Murphy, M., Sunnerhagen, K. S., Johnels, B., & Willén, C. (2006). Three-dimensional kinematic motion analysis of a daily activity drinking from a glass: a pilot study. *Journal of Neuroengineering and Rehabilitation*, *3*(1), 18.

Amirjani, N., Ashworth, N. L., Olson, J. L., Morhart, M., & Chan, K. M. (2011). Validity and reliability of the Purdue Pegboard Test in carpal tunnel syndrome. *Muscle & Nerve*, *43*(2), 171–7.

Ávila, R., Bottino, C. M. C., Carvalho, I. A. M., Santos, C. B., Seral, C., & Miotto, E. C. (2004). Neuropsychological rehabilitation of memory deficits and activities of daily living in patients with Alzheimer's disease : a pilot study. *Brazilian Journal of Medical and Biological Research*, *37*, 1721–1729. doi:10.1590/S0100-879X2004001100018

Backman, C., & Mackie, H. (1995). Arthritis hand function test: inter-rater reliability among self-trained raters. *Arthritis Care and Research : The Official Journal of the Arthritis Health Professions Association*, *8*(1), 10–5.

Bartolo, M., Zucchella, C., Pace, A., Lanzetta, G., Vecchione, C., Bartolo, M., … Pierelli, F. (2012). Early rehabilitation after surgery improves functional outcome in inpatients with brain tumours. *Journal of Neuro-Oncology*, *107*(3), 537–44.

Bendstrup, K. E., Ingemann Jensen, J., Holm, S., & Bengtsson, B. (1997). Out-patient rehabilitation improves activities of daily living, quality of life and exercise tolerance in chronic obstructive pulmonary disease. *European Respiratory Journal*, *10*, 2801–2806. doi:10.1183/09031936.97.10122801

Bendstrup, K., Ingemann Jensen, J., Holm, S., & Bengtsson, B. (1997). Out-patient rehabilitation improves activities of daily living, quality of life and exercise tolerance in chronic obstructive pulmonary disease. *Eur. Respir. J.*, *10*(12), 2801–2806.

Bohannon, R. W. (2001). Dynamometer measurements of hand-grip strength predict multiple outcomes. *Perceptual and Motor Skills*, *93*, 323–328. doi:10.2466/pms.2001.93.2.323

Bohannon, R. W., Peolsson, A., Massy-Westropp, N., Desrosiers, J., & Bear-Lehman, J. (2006). Reference values for adult grip strength measured with a Jamar dynamometer: a descriptive meta-analysis. *Physiotherapy*, *92*(1), 11–15.

Brogardh, C., Persson, A. L., & Sjolund, B. H. (2007). Intra- and inter-rater reliability of the Sollerman hand function test in patients with chronic stroke. *Disability and Rehabilitation*.

Bullock, I. M., Zheng, J. Z., Rosa, S. D. La, Guertler, C., & Dollar, A. M. (2013). Grasp Frequency and Usage in Daily Household and Machine Shop Tasks. *IEEE Transactions on Haptics*, *6*(3), 296–308. doi:10.1109/TOH.2013.6

Butler, E. E., Ladd, A. L., Louie, S. A., Lamont, L. E., Wong, W., & Rose, J. (2010). Three-dimensional kinematics of the upper limb during a Reach and Grasp Cycle for children. *Gait & Posture*, *32*(1), 72–7.

Cano-de la Cuerda, R., Águila-Maturana, A. M., & Macías-Jiménez, A. I. (2008). Valoración manual de la fuerza muscular frente a dinamometría instrumental. *Rehabilitación*, *42*(5), 260–261. doi:10.1016/S0048-7120(08)74602-4.

Changulani, M., Okonkwo, U., Keswani, T., & Kalairajah, Y. (2008). Outcome evaluation measures for wrist and hand: which one to choose? *International Orthopaedics*, *32*(1), 1–6. doi:10.1007/s00264-007-0368-z

Chemerinski, E., Robinson, R. G., & Kosier, J. T. (2001). Improved Recovery in Activities of Daily Living Associated With Remission of Poststroke Depression. *Stroke*, *32*(1), 113–117.

Chen, W., Xiong, C., Huang, X., Sun, R., & Xiong, Y. (2010). Kinematic analysis and dexterity evaluation of upper extremity in activities of daily living. *Gait & Posture*, *32*(4), 475–81.

Chiou, I. I., & Burnett, C. N. (1985). Values of activities of daily living. A survey of stroke patients and their home therapists. *Physical Therapy*, *65*, 901–906.

Connell, L. A., McMahon, N. E., Watkins, C. L., & Eng, J. J. (2014). Therapists' use of the Graded Repetitive Arm Supplementary Program (GRASP) intervention: a practice implementation survey study. *Physical Therapy*, *94*(5), 632–43.

Coster, W., Haley, S. M., Jette, A., Tao, W., & Siebens, H. (2007). Predictors of Basic and Instrumental Activities of Daily Living Performance in Persons Receiving Rehabilitation Services. *Archives of Physical Medicine and Rehabilitation*, *88*, 928–935. doi:10.1016/j.apmr.2007.03.037

De Carvalho, R. M. F., Mazzer, N., & Barbieri, C. H. (2012). Analysis of the reliability and reproducibility of goniometry compared to hand photogrammetry. *Acta Ortopedica Brasileira*, *20*(3), 139–49. doi:10.1590/S1413-78522012000300003

De Smet, L., De Kesel, R., Degreef, I., & Debeer, P. (2007). Responsiveness of the Dutch version of the DASH as an outcome measure for carpal tunnel syndrome. *The Journal of Hand Surgery, European Volume*, *32*(1), 74–6. doi:10.1016/j.jhsb.2006.10.001

Deloitte Access Economics. (2011). *The economic benefits of increasing employment for people with disability*. Commissioned by the Australian Network on Disability. August.

Demers, L., Desrosiers, J., Nikolova, R., Robichaud, L., & Bravo, G. (2010). Responsiveness of Mobility, Daily Living, and Instrumental Activities of Daily Living Outcome Measures for Geriatric Rehabilitation. *Archives of Physical Medicine and Rehabilitation*, *91*, 233–240. doi:10.1016/j.apmr.2009.10.007

Ellis, B., & Bruton, A. (2002). A study to compare the reliability of composite finger flexion with goniometry for measurement of range of motion in the hand. *Clinical Rehabilitation*, *16*(5), 562–570.

Engelberg, A. L. (1988). *Guides to the evaluation of permanent impairment*. American Medical Association.

Engstrand, C., Krevers, B., & Kvist, J. (2011). Interrater Reliability in Finger Joint Goniometer Measurement in Dupuytren's Disease. *American Journal of Occupational Therapy*, *66*(1), 98–103.

Faria-Fortini, I., Michaelsen, S. M., Cassiano, J. G., & Teixeira-Salmela, L. F. (2011). Upper extremity function in stroke subjects: relationships between the international classification of functioning, disability, and health domains. *Journal of Hand Therapy : Official Journal of the American Society of Hand Therapists*, *24*(3), 257–64; quiz 265.

Grao, C., Cervera, J., Maez, I., Viosca, E., Almagro, P., & Gonzalez, C. (2006). Escalas de valoración funcional de la mano. Revisión bibliográfica. *Communication Hospital LaFe Valencia.*

Guidali, M., Duschau-Wicke, A., Broggi, S., Klamroth-Marganska, V., Nef, T., & Riener, R. (2011). A robotic system to train activities of daily living in a virtual environment. *Medical and Biological Engineering and Computing*, *49*, 1213–1223. doi:10.1007/s11517-011-0809-0.

Hellström, K., Lindmark, B., Wahlberg, B., & Fugl-Meyer, A. R. (2003). Self-efficacy in relation to impairments and activities of daily living disability in elderly patients with stroke: A prospective investigation. *Journal of Rehabilitation Medicine*, *35*, 202–207. doi:10.1080/16501970310000836

Hemmerich, A., Brown, H., Smith, S., Marthandam, S. S. K., & Wyss, U. P. (2006). Hip, knee, and ankle kinematics of high range of motion activities of daily living. *Journal of Orthopaedic Research : Official Publication of the Orthopaedic Research Society*, *24*(4), 770–81. doi:10.1002/jor.20114

Henmi, S., Yonenobu, K., Masatomi, T., & Oda, K. (2006). A biomechanical study of activities of daily living using neck and upper limbs with an optical three-dimensional motion analysis system. *Modern Rheumatology/the Japan Rheumatism Association*, *16*(5), 289–93. doi:10.1007/s10165-006-0499-x

Hernandez-Milagro, M. A., Rodríguez-García, G. T., & Gerona-Galdame, P. (2008). La discapacidad en España. Equipos de valoración y orientación (EVO). Prestaciones. Valoración de la discapacidad por disfunción del sistema musculoesquelético y nervioso | Rehabilitación. *Rehabilitación, Vol. 42(6)*, 276–86.

Holmes, E. B. (2013). Impairment Rating and Disability Determination. *Medscape*.

Hudak, P. L., Amadio, P. C., & Bombardier, C. (2008). The DASH questionnaire and score in the evaluation of hand and wrist disorders. *Acta Orthopaedica Belgica*, *74*(5), 575–581. doi:10.1002/(SICI)1097-0274(199606)29:6<602::AID-AJIM4>3.0.CO;2-L

Hume, M. C., Gellman, H., McKellop, H., & Brumfield, R. H. (1990). Functional range of motion of the joints of the hand. *The Journal of Hand Surgery*, *15*(2), 240–243. doi:10.1016/0363-5023(90)90102-W

Jefatura del Estado España. Ley 39/2006, de 14 de diciembre, de Promoción de la Autonomía Personal y Atención a las personas en situación de dependencia (2006).

Kempen, G. I. J. M., Ballemans, J., Ranchor, A. V., Van Rens, G. H. M. B., & Zijlstra, G. A. R. (2012). The impact of low vision on activities of daily living, symptoms of depression, feelings of anxiety and social support in community-living older adults seeking vision rehabilitation services. *Quality of Life Research*, *21*, 1405–1411. doi:10.1007/s11136-011-0061-y

Kilbreath, S. L., & Heard, R. C. (2005). Frequency of hand use in healthy older persons. *Australian Journal of Physiotherapy*, *51*(2), 119–122.

Lee, J. H., Ku, J., Cho, W., Hahn, W. Y., Kim, I. Y., Lee, S.-M., … Kim, S. I. (2003). A virtual reality system for the assessment and rehabilitation of the activities of daily living. *Cyberpsychology & Behavior : The Impact of the Internet, Multimedia and Virtual Reality on Behavior and Society*, *6*, 383–388. doi:10.1089/109493103322278763

Lemmens, R. J. M., Timmermans, A. A. A., Janssen-Potten, Y. J. M., Smeets, R. J. E. M., & Seelen, H. A. M. (2012). Valid and reliable instruments for arm-hand assessment at ICF activity level in persons with hemiplegia: a systematic review. *BMC Neurology*, *12*(1), 21.

Lin, K., Chuang, L., Wu, C., Hsieh, Y., & Chang, W. (2010). Responsiveness and validity of three dexterous function measures in stroke rehabilitation. *Journal of Rehabilitation Research and Development*, *47*(6), 563–571. doi:10.1682/JRRD.2009.09.0155

Littbrand, H., Stenvall, M., & Rosendahl, E. (2011). Applicability and effects of physical exercise on physical and cognitive functions and activities of daily living among people with dementia: a systematic review. *American Journal of Physical Medicine & Rehabilitation/Association of Academic Physiatrists*, *90*, 495–518. doi:10.1097/PHM.0b013e318214de26

Liu, K. P. Y., Chan, C. C. H., Chu, M. M. L., Ng, T. Y. L., Chu, L. W., Hui, F. S. L., Fisher, A. G. (2007). Activities of daily living performance in dementia. *Acta Neurologica Scandinavica*, *116*, 91–95. doi:10.1111 /j.1600-0404.2007.00800.x

Loeb, M. E., Eide, A. H., & Mont, D. (2008). Approaching the measurement of disability prevalence: The case of Zambia. *Alter*, *2*, 32–43. doi:10.1016/j.alter.2007.06.001

Lorenzo-Agudo, M. A., Santos-García, P., & Sánchez-Belizón, D. (2007). Determinación de los valores normales de fuerza muscular de puño y pinza en una población laboral. *Rehabilitación*, *41*(5), 220–227. doi:10.1016/S0048-7120(07)75521-4

Luker, K. R., Aguinaldo, A., Kenney, D., Cahill-Rowley, K., & Ladd, A. L. (2014). Functional task kinematics of the thumb carpometacarpal joint. *Clinical Orthopaedics and Related Research*, *472*(4), 1123–9.

Macionis, V. (2013). Is diagrammatic goniometry feasible for finger ROM evaluation and self-evaluation? *Clinical Orthopaedics and Related Research*, *471*(6), 1894–903.

Magermans, D. J., Chadwick, E. K. J., Veeger, H. E. J., & van der Helm, F. C. T. (2005). Requirements for upper extremity motions during activities of daily living. *Clinical Biomechanics (Bristol, Avon)*, *20*(6), 591–9. doi:10.1016/j.clinbiomech.2005.02.006

Mainstreaming disability in the development agenda. (2008). In *Commission for Social Development, Forty-sixth Session.*

Marshall, G. A., Rentz, D. M., Frey, M. T., Locascio, J. J., Johnson, K. A., & Sperling, R. A. (2011). Executive function and instrumental activities of daily living in mild cognitive impairment and Alzheimer's disease. *Alzheimer's & Dementia : The Journal of the Alzheimer's Association*, *7*, 300–308. doi:10.1016/j.jalz.2010.04.005

Marshall, S. C., Gray, D., Wilson, K. G., Yelle, J.-D., Hébert, P., O'Rourke, K., & Jamshidi, M. (2007). A prospective study to validate an impairment questionnaire for major trauma survivors. *American Journal of Physical Medicine & Rehabilitation/Association of Academic Physiatrists*, *86*(2), 114–24. doi:10.1097/01.phm.0000253256.11686.23

Mathiowetz, V., Weber, K., Volland, G., & Kashman, N. (1984). Reliability and validity of grip and pinch strength evaluations. *The Journal of Hand Surgery*, *9*(2), 222–226.

Mehrholz, J., Kugler, J., & Pohl, M. (2011). Water-based exercises for improving activities of daily living after stroke. *Stroke*. doi:10.1161/STROKEAHA.111.613125

Metcalf, C., Adams, J., Burridge, J., Yule, V., & Chappell, P. (2007). A review of clinical upper limb assessments within the framework of the WHO ICF. *Musculoskeletal Care*, *5*(3), 160–73.

Miller, C. P., Bible, J. E., Jegede, K. A., Whang, P. G., & Grauer, J. N. (2010). The effect of rigid cervical collar height on full, active, and functional range of motion during fifteen activities of daily living. *Spine*, *35*(26), E1546–52. doi:10.1097/BRS.0b013e3181cf6f73

Mioshi, E., Hodges, J. R., & Hornberger, M. (2013). Neural correlates of activities of daily living in frontotemporal dementia. *Journal of Geriatric Psychiatry and Neurology*, *26*, 51–7. doi:10.1177/0891988713477474

Molina Rueda, F., Rivas Montero, F. M., Pérez de Heredia Torres, M., Alguacil Diego, I. M., Molero Sánchez, A., & Miangolarra Page, J. C. (2012). Movement analysis of upper extremity hemiparesis in patients with cerebrovascular disease: a pilot study. *Neurología (Barcelona, Spain)*, *27*(6), 343–7. doi:10.1016/j.nrl.2011.12.012

Murgia, A., Kyberd, P., & Barnhill, T. (2010). The use of kinematic and parametric information to highlight lack of movement and compensation in the upper extremities during activities of daily living. *Gait & Posture*, *31*(3), 300–6. doi:10.1016/j.gaitpost.2009.11.007

Norkin, C. C., & White, D. J. (2009). *Measurement of Joint Motion: A Guide to Goniometry. Part II: Upper-extremity testing.*

Oess, N. P., Wanek, J., & Curt, A. (2012). Design and evaluation of a low-cost instrumented glove for hand function assessment. *Journal of NeuroEngineering and Rehabilitation*. doi:10.1186/1743-0003-9-2

Pérez-González, A., Sancho-Bru, J. L., Mora, M. C., Iserte, J. L., Morales, A., & León, B. E. (2012). Grasp modelling with a biomechanical model of the hand. *Computer Methods in Biomechanics and Biomedical Engineering*. doi:10.1080/10255842.2012.682156

Podobnik, J., Mihelj, M., & Munih, M. (2009). Upper limb and grasp rehabilitation and evaluation of stroke patients using HenRiE device. In *2009 Virtual Rehabilitation International Conference* (pp. 173–178). IEEE.

Rahman, H. A., Fai, Y. C., & Ming, E. S. L. (2013). Evaluation of Hand Kinematics in Upward Reaching Movement. *Journal of Medical Imaging and Health Informatics*, *3*(4), 551–554.

Rantanen, T. (1999). Midlife Hand Grip Strength as a Predictor of Old Age Disability. *JAMA*, *281*(6), 558.

Roberts, H. C., Denison, H. J., Martin, H. J., Patel, H. P., Syddall, H., Cooper, C., & Sayer, A. A. (2011). A review of the measurement of grip strength in clinical and epidemiological studies: towards a standardised approach. *Age and Ageing*, *40*(4), 423–9.

Sancho-Bru, J. L., Pérez-González, A., Vergara, M., & Giurintano, D. J. (2003). A 3D biomechanical model of the hand for power grip. *Journal of Biomechanical Engineering*, *125*, 78–83. doi:10.1115/1.1532791

Sheikhzadeh, A., Yoon, J., Pinto, V. J., & Kwon, Y. W. (2008). Three-dimensional motion of the scapula and shoulder during activities of daily living. *Journal of Shoulder and Elbow Surgery/American Shoulder and Elbow Surgeons ... [et Al.]*, *17*(6), 936–42.

Soler, P. A., & Rizos, L. R. (2006). Innovaci??n en valoraci??n funcional. *Revista Espanola de Geriatria Y Gerontologia*. doi:10.1016/S0211-139X(06)72996-1

Sollerman, C., & Ejeskar, A. (1995). Sollerman hand function test: A standardised method and its use in tetraplegic patients. *Scandinavian Journal of Plastic and Reconstructive Surgery and Hand Surgery*, *29*(2), 167–176.

Stenvall, M., Olofsson, B., Nyberg, L., Lundström, M., & Gustafson, Y. (2007). Improved performance in activities of daily living and mobility after a multidisciplinary postoperative rehabilitation in older people with femoral neck fracture: A randomized controlled trial with 1-year follow-up. *Journal of Rehabilitation Medicine*, *39*, 232–238. doi:10.2340 /16501977-0045

UnitedNations. Convention on the Rights of Persons with Disabilities. , http://www.un.org/disabilities/default.asp?navid=15&pid=150 (2006).

Urwin, S., Kader, D., Caplan, N., St Clair Gibson, A., & Stewart, S. (2013, February 15). Validation of an electrogoniometry system as a measure of knee kinematics during activities of daily living. *Journal of Musculoskeletal Research*. World Scientific.

Van Andel, C. J., Wolterbeek, N., Doorenbosch, C. A. M., Veeger, D. H. E. J., & Harlaar, J. (2008). Complete 3D kinematics of upper extremity functional tasks. *Gait & Posture*, *27*(1), 120–7.

Vergara, M., Sancho-Bru, J. L., Gracia-Ibáñez, V., & Pérez-González, A. (2014). An introductory study of common grasps used by adults during performance of activities of daily living. *Journal of Hand Therapy : Official Journal of the American Society of Hand Therapists*. doi:10.1016/j.jht.2014.04.002

Wade, E., Chen, C., & Winstein, C. J. (2014). Spectral analyses of wrist motion in individuals poststroke: the development of a performance measure with promise for unsupervised settings. *Neurorehabilitation and Neural Repair*, *28*(2), 169–78.

WHO. International Classification of Functioning, Disability and Health (ICF). http://www.who.int/classifications/icf/en/ (2001). World Health Organization.

WHO. International Classification of Diseases (ICD)., http://www.who.int /classifications/icd/en/ (2010). World Health Organization.

WHO. World report on disability. http://www.who.int/ disabilities/ world_report/2011/report/en/ (2011). World Health Organization.

World Health Organization. (2002). Towards a Common Language for Functioning, Disability and Health ICF. *Geneve*.

Zheng, J. Z., Rosa, S. D. La, & Dollar, A. M. (2011a). An investigation of grasp type and frequency in daily household and machine shop tasks. *2011 IEEE International Conference on Robotics and Automation*, 4169–4175. doi:10.1109/ICRA.2011.5980366

Zheng, J. Z., Rosa, S. D. La, & Dollar, A. M. (2011b). An investigation of grasp type and frequency in daily household and machine shop tasks. *2011 IEEE International Conference on Robotics and Automation*, 4169–4175. doi:10.1109/ICRA.2011.5980366

In: Activities of Daily Living (ADL)
Editor: Scott T. Lively
ISBN: 978-1-63463-913-2

Chapter 6

Rehabilitation Strategies to Promote Independence in Daily Living Tasks for People with Cognitive Impairments

Karen P. Y. Liu, Kirralee Hazeltine, Nikki Tulliani, and Katie Balderi
University of Western Sydney,
School of Science and Health, Australia

Abstract

In this chapter, rehabilitation strategies to promote independence in daily living tasks for people with cognitive impairments will be outlined. The clienteles described in this chapter include people after a stroke or brain injury, people with Parkinson's disease and mild cognitive impartment or dementia.

Two case reports using self-regulation and mental imagery respectively, one randomized clinical trial evaluating the effectiveness of a one-week self-regulation program and two randomized clinical trials on testing the efficacy of the three-week self-regulation and mental imagery interventions on post-stroke patients will be summarized in this paper. Mental imagery has been extended to be used by people with mild cognitive impairments. The strategy helps the people to maintain a perceptual map within which the daily tasks are structured. A clinical trial using rehabilitation strategies including mental imagery to promote cognitive function necessary for daily living task performance will be summarized in this chapter. The use of external aids is common for people with Parkinson's disease to help them in initiating motor performance. This treatment strategy is believed to arouse attention of the people in starting off the motor tasks. The use of external aids and how it is internalized using the treatment technique of mental imagery will be described.

With the use of various rehabilitation strategies in the occupational therapy programs, people with cognitive impairment showed better performance of daily living tasks.

People with a neurological condition such as stroke, brain injury, Parkinson's disease (PD) or dementia might suffer from cognitive impairments which impact on their independence in activities of daily living (ADLs). For example, a study on 149 people after stroke found that 72% of the sample suffered from cognitive impairments of various kinds (Claesson, Lindén, Skoog, & Blomstrand, 2005). Their dependence in ADLs was significantly correlated with the presence of cognitive impairments.

Cognitive impairments in attention, memory, visual perception and construction were reported to be found in people after stroke (Hochstenbach & Mulder, 2003; Nys et al., 2006). For people with traumatic brain injuries, cognitive deficits are common and could include memory disturbance, reduced attention, orientation problems, word-finding difficulties (Christensen et al., 2008; Wilson, Pettigrew, & Teasdale, 2000). Cognitive impairments are being more recognized for people with PD (Bruck, Kurki, Kaasinen, Vahlberg, & Rinne, 2004; Mitchell, Kemp, Benito-León, & Reuber, 2010). Their memory and visuospatial function are affected. Among all, executive performance is more seriously affected. For people with dementia, there are numerous reports on the cognitive profile and the impairments in memory, orientation and constructional ability (Liu et al., 2011; Morris, Mohs, Rogers, Fillenbaum, & Heyman, 1988).

Rehabilitation strategies for remediating the effects of cognitive impairments on independence in ADL's include, memory training and cognitive stimulation for people with dementia (Liberati, Raffone, & Olivetti Belardinelli, 2012); memory and ADL training using external cues and internal strategies to facilitate memory performance (Ávila et al., 2004; Lim et al., 2012), attention process training (Barker-Collo et al., 2009) and cognitive skills remediation training (Carter, Howard, & O'Neil, 1983) for people with stroke (Hoffmann, Bennett, Koh, & McKenna, 2010); self-awareness training for people with brain injuries (Goverover, Johnston, Toglia, & Deluca, 2007; Leung & Liu, 2011) and self-regulation for people with stroke (Liu & Chan, 2014; Liu, Chan, Lee, Li, & Hui-Chan, 2002), mental imagery for people with stroke (Kho, Liu, & Chung, 2013; Liu, 2009; Liu, Chan, Lee, & Hui-Chan, 2004a, 2004b; Liu et al., 2009); functional training using imagery (Tamir, Dickstein, & Huberman, 2007) and external cues for people with Parkinson's disease (Akamatsu, Fukuyama, & Kawamata, 2008; Baker, Rochester, & Nieuwboer, 2007; Mak & Hui-Chan, 2008).

In the following section, two case reports using self-regulation and mental imagery, one randomized clinical trial evaluating the effectiveness of the self-regulation program and two randomized clinical trials on testing the efficacy of the combined self-regulation and mental imagery interventions on post-stroke patients are summarized. They are followed by reporting on a pilot study investigating the effectiveness of a cognitive training program that involved the use of mental imagery for people with mild cognitive impairments. The use of external cues in combination with imagery is also described.

Self-Regulation

Self-awareness of one's own problems is reported to enhance rehabilitation outcomes for people with brain injuries (Fleming & Ownsworth, 2006; Goverover et al., 2007; Leung & Liu, 2011; Liu & Chan, 2014). Requiring self-awareness to identify one's own problems, self-regulation (SR) describes reflective learning and problem solving, by bringing problems and solutions to the conscious level, in order to identify the best suitable solutions to one's problem (Gourgey, 1998). It also requires reflection on one's performance and experiences. SR refers to the ability to identify information, problem solve, anticipate problems, find solutions and internally motivate oneself, as well as reflect on one's performance and experiences (Gourgey, 1998; Leung & Liu, 2011; Liu et al., 2002; Ownsworth & Clare, 2006; Toglia & Kirk, 2000). It is an executive functioning skill controlled by the frontal lobe of the brain (Goverover et al., 2007; Ownsworth & Fleming, 2005).

A pilot study of a one-week intervention program using self-regulation to train task performance of people after stroke showed a preliminary result that

SR is able to enhance ADL functioning after stroke (Liu & Chan, 2014; Liu et al., 2002). In our studies, the one-week intervention involved training of five daily tasks. Occupational therapists used self-regulation strategies to guide the patients to identify problems when they performed those tasks. Patients were then prompted to generate possible solutions to the problems identified. During the practice of the tasks using the possible solutions, the performance is video-taped and played back to the patients. Patients would actively participate to decide on the best solution and continue to practice them. They were also guided to evaluate the problem identified, solutions generated and their performance. Results showed that self-regulation strategies could help people with stroke to learn the task at a metacognitive level. They do so by approaching the tasks strategically, understanding the effective problem-solving procedures, checking on their own performance and reflecting on their success. As illustrated in the case report (Liu et al., 2002) and the randomized clinical trial (Liu & Chan, 2014), through active learning, people with different impairments resulting from a lesion in different sites of the brain would benefit from the use of self-regulation to enhance their relearning of ADL's.

Mental Imagery

Mental imagery is a process in which behavior is rehearsed mentally as if the person is actually performing it. It is believed to enhance relearning by involving people in actively gathering perceptual information from memory and undergoing the experience of "seeing the performance of the behaviour with the mind's eye" (Kosslyn, Ganis, & Thompson, 2001). Numerous researches have proven the effectiveness of mental imagery to enhance function for people with cognitive impairments. For example, it enhances relearning of ADLs, maintaining the tasks learnt and generalizing to new tasks and new environments (Liu, 2009; Liu et al., 2004a, 2004b; Liu et al., 2009); improves upper extremity function (Kho et al., 2013; Page, Levine, & Leonard, 2005), promotes sit-to-stand and reaching abilities (Guttman, Burstin, Brown, Bril, & Dickstein, 2012), and improves gait for people with stroke (Verma, Arya, Garg, & Singh, 2011); improves memory (Potvin, Rouleau, Senechal, & Giguere, 2011), enhances work tasks sequencing for people with executive functioning impairment (Precin, 2010), and promotes elbow extension in patients with quadriplegia (Grangeon et al., 2010). The following section describes the evidence of a three-week mental imagery program to promote relearning and generalization for people with stroke.

For People with Stroke

A case report showed mental imagery was effective at improving the relearning of function for people with stroke (Liu et al., 2004b). Mental imagery has the potential to increase a person's task performance which does not require significantly high motor functions but is cognitively complicated to perform. A series of follow-up studies were completed to investigate the effectiveness of the mental imagery program using a randomized controlled trial (RCT) design. The mental imagery program consists of three weeks of training with five sessions each week. Fifteen daily tasks with appropriate motor and cognitive demands were included. Patients were trained with five tasks each week using the technique of mental imagery. Mental imagery and actual task performance were practiced each week to help the patients to develop competence in utilizing imagery as a learning tool and transforming imagery into real task performance. Patients were engaged into imagery to identify their own problems for rectification. They were then asked to practice the rectified task performance using both imagery and actual practice. Visual aids were used to facilitate the patients to reflect on the problems that they encountered when they actually performed the tasks. They watched the video playback to confirm the problems that they identified and were guided to develop strategies to overcome the problems. The tasks, with or without modifications, were mentally imagined before the patients practiced them. Mental imagery and actual practice went on throughout the process. Results of a RCT (Liu et al., 2004a) showed that mental imagery would be an effective training strategy to promote the relearning and generalization of daily tasks for people after an acute stroke. Another RCT conducted, provides further indication that mental imagery enhanced the generalization of skills learnt to tasks in a new environment (Liu, 2009; Liu et al., 2009). The results of these studies demonstrated that mental imagery, not only enhanced one's relearning of task performance, but promoted generalization of skills learnt to new tasks and in new environments. The ability to generalize skills learnt is important for patients to be able to cope with their daily tasks after discharge from the hospital to home environment. The imagery process in the 3-week mental imagery program was postulated to improve the planning and execution of tasks, and in turn assist people in anticipating the task demands and therefore enhancing task performance.

For People with Mild Cognitive Impairments or Dementia

Imagery techniques have been reported 30 years ago to alleviate memory loss for people with dementia (for example, Jean, Bergeron, Thivierge, & Simard, 2010; Tardif & Simard, 2011; Zarit, Zarit, & Reever, 1982). A recent study using multifaceted cognitive training for people with mild cognitive impairments also adopted imagery in the training (Lim et al., 2012). Method of loci is one way to adopt imagery to help a person remember things (Lim et al., 2012). The process involves a person imagining the stimulus to be remembered and placing it in a predetermined spatial context. By imaging a task in a familiar spatial context such as their own home, the individual can recall the task sequence and the task performance could be enhanced. The effective use of strategies could encourage a person to perform deeper analysis and elaborative encoding of the material to be recalled which enhances retrieval (Allan, Robb, & Rugg, 2000; Kuo, Liu, & Chan, 2012; Kuo, Liu, Ting, & Chan, 2012).

External Cues and Imagery

For People with Parkinson's Disease

The use of external cues as a rehabilitation strategy to improve gait performance of people with PD was first reported in 1942 (Von Wilzelben, 1942). Studies further investigating the effect of external cues are being conducted. Both experimental and clinical studies show that external cues can diminish the bradykinesia symptom of people with PD (for example, Arias & Cudeiro, 2010; Katherine Baker, Rochester, & Nieuwboer, 2008; Kadivar, Corcos, Foto, & Hondzinski, 2011; Nieuwboer et al., 2007; Rochester et al., 2010; Rochester et al., 2007). External cues are described as using spatial or temporal stimuli, including all kinds of sensory stimulation, to facilitate the motor function for people with motor dysfunction. Three types of external cues are defined here based on the sensory stimulation involved. They include visual cue, auditory cue, and tactile cue. Examples include the auditory cue of a rhythmic metronome, the visual cue of a flashing light, and the tactile cue of a vibration on body parts (Marchese, Diverio, Zucchi, Lentino, & Abbruzzese, 2000; Nieuwboer et al., 2009). Studies demonstrate the effectiveness of external cues on gait (for example, M. E. Morris, Iansek, Matyas, & Summers, 1996), reaching movements (for example, Kelly, Hyngstrom, Rundle, & Bastian, 2002; Majsak, Kaminski, Gentile, & Flanagan, 1998), and complex functional performance such as driving (Scally et al., 2011; Stolwyk, Triggs, Charlton, Iansek, & Bradshaw, 2005).

A recent study has reported the use of mental imagery for people with PD (Tamir et al., 2007). The imagery program used in the study aimed at improving the smooth performance of movement sequences such as standing up and sitting down. It was combined with the use of external cues. Although evidence has shown that the imagery ability of people with PD is preserved (Heremans et al., 2011), adding external cues to imagery was shown to enhance the imagery quality of people with PD, that might in turn promote the efficacy of using imagery to enhance their function (Heremans et al., 2012). However, further research is needed to investigate the effects and mechanism of imagery in enhancing function for people with PD.

Conclusion

Cognitive engagement and stimulation are known to modify the brain processes to perform tasks by recruiting alternative and more efficient neural networks (Kuo, Liu, Ting, & Chan, 2014; Kuo et al., 2014; Kuo, Liu, & Chan, 2012; Kuo, Liu, Ting, et al., 2012). Treatment strategies to promote improvement in ADLs and function for people with cognitive impairments could gear towards engaging the person in cognitive tasks or providing stimulation. In this chapter, the use of self-regulation and mental imagery for people with different diagnoses who might experience cognitive impairments are reported. In conclusion, rehabilitation strategies that gradually build on skills learnt, enhance deeper analysis and elaborative encoding of the material would be beneficial and potentially enhance one's functioning (Kuo, Liu, & Chan, 2012; Liu, Chan, Tulliani, Ng, & Li, 2014). Further research is needed to investigate the use of these strategies across different diagnostic groups in various contexts. The study of the underlying mechanism on how the strategies work would also warrant further investigation.

Acknowledgments

This book chapter was partly supported by the School of Science and Health Research Grants 2013 and 2014 from University of Western Sydney awarded to K.P.Y. Liu.

References

Akamatsu, T., Fukuyama, H., & Kawamata, T. (2008). The effects of visual, auditory, and mixed cues on choice reaction in Parkinson's disease. *Journal of the Neurological Sciences, 269*, 118-125.

Allan, K., Robb, W. G. K., & Rugg, M. D. (2000). The effect of encoding manipulations on neural correlates of episodic retrieval. *Neuropsychologia, 38*, 1188-1205.

Arias, P., & Cudeiro, J. (2010). Effect of Rhythmic Auditory Stimulation on Gait in Parkinsonian Patients with and without Freezing of Gait. *PLoS ONE, 5*(3), e9675. doi: 10.1371/journal.pone.0009675

Ávila, R., Bottino, C. M. C., Carvalho, I. A. M., Santos, C. B., Seral, C., & Miotto, E. C. (2004). Neuropsychological rehabilitation of memory deficits and activities of daily living in patients with Alzheimer's disease: A pilot study. *Brazilian Journal of Medical and Biological Research, 37*, 1721-1729.

Baker, K., Rochester, L., & Nieuwboer, A. (2007). The immediate effect of attentional, auditory, and a combined cue strategy on gait during single and dual tasks in Parkinson's disease. *Archives of Physical Medicine and Rehabilitation, 88*, 1593-1600.

Baker, K., Rochester, L., & Nieuwboer, A. (2008). The effect of cues on gait variability—Reducing the attentional cost of walking in people with Parkinson's disease. *Parkinsonism & Related Disorders, 14*(4), 314-320. doi: 10.1016/j.parkreldis.2007.09.008

Barker-Collo, S. L., Feigin, V. L., Lawes, C. M., Parag, V., Senior, H., & Rodgers, A. (2009). Reducing attention deficits after stroke using attention process training: a randomized controlled trial. *Stroke*(10), 3293-3298.

Bruck, A., Kurki, T., Kaasinen, V., Vahlberg, T., & Rinne, J. O. (2004). Hippocampal and prefrontal atrophy in patients with early non-demented Parkinson's disease is related to cognitive impairment. *Journal of Neurology, Neurosurgery and Psychiatry, 75*, 1467-1469.

Carter, L. T., Howard, B. E., & O'Neil, W. A. (1983). Effectiveness of cognitive skill remediation in acute stroke patients. *American Journal of Occupational Therapy, 37*, 320-326.

Christensen, B. K., Colella, B., Inness, E., Hebert, D., Monette, G., Bayley, M., & Green, R. E. (2008). Recovery of cognitive function after traumatic brain injury: a multilevel modeling analysis of canadian outcomes. *Archives of Physical Medicine and Rehabilitation, 89*, S3-S15.

Claesson, L., Lindén, T., Skoog, I., & Blomstrand, C. (2005). Cognitive impairment after stroke – Impact on activities of daily living and costs of care for elderly people. *Cerebrovascular Diseases, 19*, 102-109.

Fleming, J. M., & Ownsworth, T. (2006). A review of awareness interventions in brain injury rehabilitation. *Neuropsychological Rehabilitation, 16*, 474-500.

Gourgey, A. F. (1998). Metacognition in basic skills instruction. *Instructional Sciences, 26*, 81-96.

Goverover, Y., Johnston, M. V., Toglia, J., & Deluca, J. (2007). Treatment to improve self-awareness in persons with acquired brain injury. *Brain Injury, 21*, 913-923.

Grangeon, M., Guillot, A., Sancho, P. O., Picot, M., Revol, P., Rode, G., & Collet, C. (2010). Rehabilitation of the elbow extension with motor imagery in a patient with quadriplegia after tendon transfer. *Archives of Physical Medicine & Rehabilitation, 91*, 1143-1146.

Guttman, A., Burstin, A., Brown, R., Bril, S., & Dickstein, R. (2012). Motor imagery practice for improving sit to stand and reaching to grasp in individuals with poststroke hemiparesis. *Topics in Stroke Rehabilitation, 19*, 306-319.

Heremans, E., Feys, P., Nieuwboer, A., Vercruysse, S., Vandenberghe, W., Sharma, N., & Helsen, W. (2011). Motor imagery ability in patients with early- and mid-stage Parkinson disease. *Neurorehabilitation and Neural Repair, 25*, 168-177.

Heremans, E., Nieuwboer, A., Feys, P., Vercruysse, S., Vandenberghe, W., Sharma, N., & Helsen, W. F. (2012). External cueing improves motor imagery quality in patients with Parkinson disease. *Neurorehabilitation & Neural Repair, 26*, 27-35.

Hochstenbach, J. B., & Mulder, T. W. (2003). Cognitive recovery after stroke: a 2-year follow-up. *Archives of Physical Medicine and Rehabilitation, 84*, 1499-1504.

Hoffmann, T., Bennett, S., Koh, C.-L., & McKenna, K. (2010). A systematic review of cognitive interventions to improve functional ability in people who have cognitive impairment following stroke.Detail Only Available Hoffmann, Tammy Bennett, Sally Koh, Chia-Lin McKenna, Kryss ; Topics in Stroke Rehabilitation, Vol 17(2), Mar-Apr, 2010. pp. 99-107. *Topics in Stroke Rehabilitation, 17*, 99-107.

Jean, L., Bergeron, M., Thivierge, S., & Simard, M. (2010). Cognitive intervention programs for individuals with mild cognitive impairment: Systematic review of the literature. *American Journal of Geriatric Psychiatry, 18*, 281-296.

Kadivar, Z., Corcos, D. M., Foto, J., & Hondzinski, J. M. (2011). Effect of Step Training and Rhythmic Auditory Stimulation on Functional Performance in Parkinson Patients. *Neurorehabilitation and Neural Repair, 25*(7), 626-635. doi: 10.1177/1545968311401627

Kelly, V. E., Hyngstrom, A. S., Rundle, M. M., & Bastian, A. J. (2002). Interaction of levodopa and cues on voluntary reaching in Parkinson's disease. *Movement Disorders, 17*, 38-44.

Kho, A. Y., Liu, K. P. Y., & Chung, R. C. K. (2013). Meta-analysis on the effect of mental imagery on motor recovery of the hemiplegic upper extremity function. *Australian Occupational Therapy Journal*. doi: doi: 10.1111/1440-1630.12084

Kosslyn, S. M., Ganis, G., & Thompson, W. L. (2001). Neural foundations of imagery. *Nature Reviews Neuroscience, 2*, 635-642.

Kuo, C. C. M., Liu, K. P. Y., Ting, K.-H., & Chan, C. C. H. (2014). Age-related Effects on Perceptual and Semantic Encoding in Memory. *Neuroscience, 261*, 95-106.

Kuo, M. C. C., Liu, K. P. Y., Bissett, M., Wesson, J., Tulliani, N., & Bye, R. (2014). Memory Encoding Processes in Younger and Older Adults. *Archives of Neuroscience, 2*, e19813.

Kuo, M. C. C., Liu, K. P. Y., & Chan, C. C. H. (2012). Factors modulating memory encoding and their implications for the memory performance of older adults and people with mild cognitive impairment: A critical review. *World Journal of Neuroscience, 2*(2), 103-112.

Kuo, M. C. C., Liu, K. P. Y., Ting, K.-H., & Chan, C. C. H. (2012). Differentiation of perceptual and semantic subsequent memory effects using an orthographic paradigm. *Brain Research, 1486*, 82-91. doi: 10.1016/j.brainres.2012.10.005

Leung, D. P. K., & Liu, K. P. Y. (2011). Review of Self-Awareness and its Clinical Application in Stroke Rehabilitation. *International Journal of Rehabilitation Research, 34*, 187-195.

Liberati, G., Raffone, A., & Olivetti Belardinelli, M. (2012). Cognitive reserve and its implications for rehabilitation and Alzheimer's disease. *Cognitive Processing, 13*, 1-12.

Lim, M. H. X., Liu, K. P. Y., Cheung, G. S. F., Kuo, M. C. C., Li, R., & Tong, C.-Y. (2012). A Multifaceted Cognitive Training Programme for People with Mild Cognitive Impairment. *Hong Kong Journal of Occupational Therapy, 22*, 3-8. doi: 10.1016/j.hkjot.2012.04.002.

Liu, K. P. Y. (2009). Use of mental imagery to improve task generalisation after a stroke. *Hong Kong Medical Journal, 15*, 37-41.

Liu, K. P. Y., & Chan, C. C. H. (2014). A pilot randomized controlled trial of self-regulation in promoting function in acute post-stroke patients. *Archives of Physical Medicine and Rehabilitation, 95*, 1262-1267.

Liu, K. P. Y., Chan, C. C. H., Lee, T. M. C., & Hui-Chan, C. W. Y. (2004a). Mental Imagery for Promoting Relearning for People After Stroke: A Randomized Controlled Trial. *Archives of Physical Medicine and Rehabilitation, 85*, 1403-1408.

Liu, K. P. Y., Chan, C. C. H., Lee, T. M. C., & Hui-Chan, C. W. Y. (2004b). Mental Imagery for Relearning of People after Brain Injury. *Brain Injury, 18*, 1163-1172.

Liu, K. P. Y., Chan, C. C. H., Lee, T. M. C., Li, L. S. W., & Hui-Chan, C. W. Y. (2002). Case Reports on Self-regulatory Learning and Generalization for People with Brain Injury. *Brain Injury, 16*, 817-824.

Liu, K. P. Y., Chan, C. C. H., Tulliani, N., Ng, M. C. K., & Li, L. S. W. (2014). Rehabilitation programme to promote task relearning and generalisation after stroke: A review of literature. *Journal of Neurology and Neurophysiology, 5*(4), 1000220.

Liu, K. P. Y., Chan, C. C. H., Wong, R. S. M., Kwan, I. W. L., Yau, C. S. F., Li, L. S. W., & Lee, T. M. C. (2009). A randomized controlled trial of mental imagery augment generalization of learning in acute poststroke patients. *Stroke, 40*, 2222-2225.

Liu, K. P. Y., Kuo, M. C. C., Tang, K.-C., Chau, A. W. S., Ho, I. H. T., Kwok, M. P. H., . . . Chu, L. W. (2011). Effects of age, education and gender in the Consortium to Establish a Registry for the Alzheimer's Disease (CERAD)-Neuropsychological Assessment Battery for Cantonese-speaking Chinese Elders. *International Psychogeriatrics, 23*, 1575-1581.

Majsak, M. J., Kaminski, T., Gentile, A. M., & Flanagan, J. R. (1998). The reaching movements of patients with Parkinson's disease under self-determined maximal speed and visually cued conditions. *Brain, 121*, 755-766.

Mak, M. K., & Hui-Chan, C. W. (2008). Cued task-specific training is better than exercise in improving sit-to-stand in patients with Parkinson's disease: A randomized controlled trial. *Movement Disorders, 23*, 501-509.

Marchese, R., Diverio, M., Zucchi, F., Lentino, C., & Abbruzzese, G. (2000). The role of sensory cues in the rehabilitation of parkinsonian patients: A comparison of two physical therapy protocols. *Movement Disorders, 15*(5), 879-883. doi: 10.1002/1531-8257(200009)15:5<879::aid-mds1018>3.0.co;2-9

Mitchell, A. J., Kemp, S., Benito-León, J., & Reuber, M. (2010). The influence of cognitive impairment on health-related quality of life in neurological disease. *Acta Neuropsychiatrica, 22*, 2-13.

Morris, J. C., Mohs, R. C., Rogers, H., Fillenbaum, G., & Heyman, A. (1988). Consortium to establish a registry for Alzheimer's disease (CERAD). Clinical and neuropsychological assessment of Alzheimer's disease. *Psychopharmacology Bulletin, 24*, 641-652.

Morris, M. E., Iansek, R., Matyas, T. A., & Summers, J. J. (1996). Stride length regulation in Parkinson's disease. Normalization strategies and underlying mechanisms. *Brain, 119*, 551-568.

Nieuwboer, A., Baker, K., Willems, A.-M., Jones, D., Spildooren, J., Lim, I., Rochester, L. (2009). The Short-Term Effects of Different Cueing Modalities on Turn Speed in People with Parkinson's Disease. *Neurorehabilitation and Neural Repair, 23*(8), 831-836. doi: 10.1177/1545968309337136

Nieuwboer, A., Kwakkel, G., Rochester, L., Jones, D., van Wegen, E., Willems, A. M., Lim, I. (2007). Cueing training in the home improves gait-related mobility in Parkinson's disease: the RESCUE trial. *Journal of Neurology, Neurosurgery & Psychiatry, 78*(2), 134-140. doi: 10.1136/jnnp.200X.097923

Nys, G. M., van Zandvoort, M. J., van der Worp, H. B., de Haan, E. H., de Kort, P. L., Jansen, B. P., & Kappelle, L. J. (2006). Early cognitive impairment predicts long-term depressive symptoms and quality of life after stroke. *Journal of the Neurological Sciences, 247*, 149-156.

Ownsworth, T., & Clare, L. (2006). The association between awareness deficits and rehabilitation outcome following acquired brain injury. *Clinical Psychology Review, 26*, 783-795.

Ownsworth, T., & Fleming, J. (2005). The Relative Importance of Metacognitive Skills, Emotional Status, and Executive Function in Psychosocial Adjustment Following Acquired Brain Injury. *The Journal of Head Trauma Rehabilitation, 20*, 315-332.

Page, S. J., Levine, P., & Leonard, A. C. (2005). Effects of mental practice on affected limb use and function in chronic stroke. *Archives of Physical Medicine and Rehabilitation, 86*, 399-402.

Potvin, M. J., Rouleau, I., Senechal, G., & Giguere, J. F. (2011). Prospective memory rehabilitation based on visual imagery techniques. *Neuropsychological Rehabilitation, 21*, 899-924.

Precin, P. (2010). The use of visual imagery to enhance sequencing of work tasks. *Work, 36*, 373-379.

Rochester, L., Baker, K., Hetherington, V., Jones, D., Willems, A.-M., Kwakkel, G., Nieuwboer, A. (2010). Evidence for motor learning in Parkinson's disease: Acquisition, automaticity and retention of cued gait performance after training with external rhythmical cues. *Brain Research, 1319*(0), 103-111. doi: 10.1016/j.brainres.2010.01.001

Rochester, L., Nieuwboer, A., Baker, K., Hetherington, V., Willems, A. M., Chavret, F., Jones, D. (2007). The attentional cost of external rhythmical cues and their impact on gait in Parkinson's disease: effect of cue modality and task complexity. *Journal of Neural Transmission, 114*(10), 1243-1248. doi: 10.1007/s00702-007-0756-y

Scally, K., Charlton, J. L., Iansek, R., Bradshaw, J. L., Moss, S., & Georgiou-Karistianis, N. (2011). Impact of External Cue Validity on Driving Performance in Parkinson's Disease. *Parkinson's Disease, 2011*. doi: 10.4061/2011/159621

Stolwyk, R. J., Triggs, T. J., Charlton, J. L., Iansek, R., & Bradshaw, J. L. (2005). Impact of internal versus external cueing on driving performance in people with Parkinson's disease. *Movement Disorders, 20*(7), 846-857. doi: 10.1002/mds.20420

Tamir, R., Dickstein, R., & Huberman, M. (2007). Integration of motor imagery and physical practice in group treatment applied to subjects with parkinson's disease. *Neurorehabilitation and Neural Repair, 21*, 68-75.

Tardif, S., & Simard, M. (2011). Cognitive stimulation programs in healthy elderly: a review. *International journal of Alzheimer's disease, 2011*. doi:10.4061/2011/378934

Toglia, J., & Kirk, U. (2000). Understanding awareness deficits following brain injury. *Neurorehabilitation, 15*, 57-70.

Verma, R., Arya, K. N., Garg, R. K., & Singh, T. (2011). Task-oriented circuit class training program with motor imagery for gait rehabilitation in poststroke patients: a randomized controlled trial. *Topics in Stroke Rehabilitation, 18* (Suppl 1), 620-632.

Von Wilzelben, H. D. (1942). *Methods in the treatment of post encephalic Parkinson's* (pp. 4).

Wilson, J. T. L., Pettigrew, L. E. L., & Teasdale, G. M. (2000). Emotional and cognitive consequences of head injury in relation to the Glasgow outcome scale. *Journal of Neurology, Neurosurgery and Psychiatry, 69*, 204-209.

Zarit, S. H., Zarit, J. M., & Reever, K. E. (1982). Memory training for severe memory loss: effects on senile dementia patients and their families. *The Gerontologist, 22*, 373-377.

Index

A

B

C

L

M

N

O

P

Q

R

S

T

U

V

W